Get Through

MRCPsych: MCQs for Paper 3

Arunraj Kaimal MBBS MRCPsych
Consultant Old Age Psychiatrist and Honorary Lecturer in Psychiatry,
Wythenshawe Hospital, Manchester, UK

Manoj Rajagopal MBBS MRCPsych MSc
ST-5 in Old Age Psychiatry, Hope Hospital, Manchester, UK

Salman Karim MBBS FCPS MSc
Consultant Old Age Psychiatrist and Honorary Lecturer in Psychiatry,
Hope Hospital, Manchester, UK

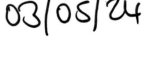

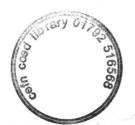

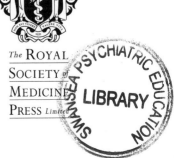

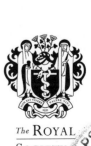

The ROYAL
SOCIETY of
MEDICINE
PRESS Limited

© 2009 Royal Society of Medicine Press Ltd

Published by the Royal Society of Medicine Press Ltd
1 Wimpole Street, London W1G 0AE, UK
Tel: +44 (0)20 7290 2921
Fax: +44 (0)20 7290 2929
Email: publishing@rsm.ac.uk
Website: www.rsmpress.co.uk

British Library Cataloguing in Publication Data
A catalogue record for this book is available from the British Library

ISBN: 978-1-85315-863-6

Distribution in Europe and Rest of World:
Marston Book Services Ltd
PO Box 269
Abingdon
Oxon OX14 4YN, UK
Tel: +44 (0)1235 465500
Fax: +44 (0)1235 465555
Email: direct.order@marston.co.uk

Distribution in the USA and Canada:
Royal Society of Medicine Press Ltd
c/o BookMasters Inc
30 Amberwood Parkway
Ashland, OH 44805, USA
Tel: +1 800 247 6553/+1 800 266 5564
Fax: +1 419 281 6883
Email: order@bookmasters.com

Distribution in Australia and New Zealand:
Elsevier Australia
30–52 Smidmore Street
Marrickville NSW 2204, Australia
Tel: +61 2 9517 8999
Fax: +61 2 9517 2249
Email: service@elsevier.com.au

Typeset by Techset Composition Limited, Salisbury, UK
Printed and bound in Great Britain by Bell & Bain, Glasgow

Contents

Introduction

The examination

The new MRCPsych examination consists of three written papers and one clinical examination (the CASC). There have been major changes to the format of the examination recently, the most important being the change from individual statement questions (ISQs) and extended matching items (EMIs) to 'best answer 1 of 5' style multiple choice questions (MCQs) and EMIs. Although there are a number of ISQ and EMI books available on the market, there are very few dedicated solely to the new-format 'best answer 1 of 5' MCQs.

In this book we have attempted to overcome this shortfall by providing 387 MCQs covering all areas of the MRCPsych Paper 3 curriculum. The questions in this book are presented according to the subheadings in the new curriculum will make revision easier, making this book an essential companion for trainees preparing for the MRCPsych Paper 3 examination.

As described in the curriculum, each MCQ comprises a question stem, which is usually one or two sentences long but may be longer. The question stem is followed by a list of five options; candidates should choose the single option that best fits the question stem.

The MRCPsych Paper 3 examination is 3 hours long and contains 200 questions. Approximately one-third of the examination will be the EMI component. Candidates are advised to attempt all questions. No marks are deducted for incorrect answers. One mark is given for the correct answer.

Revising for the examination

The topics included in the Paper 3 examination are critical appraisal, statistics, research methods and clinical management topics from general adult psychiatry and psychiatric subspecialties. Candidates' knowledge of the latest developments in these fields is tested in the Paper 3 examination and therefore candidates are advised to use the latest editions of textbooks for revision. They are also advised to be familiar with the guidelines produced by the National Institute for Health and Clinical Excellence (NICE) and the evidence base for the diagnostic and therapeutic procedures used in clinical practice. In addition to this, candidates are advised to be familiar with the topics covered in the review articles (over the 12–18-month period before the examination) in the Royal College of Psychiatrists' journal *Advances in Psychiatric Treatment*, and editorials and review articles in *The British Journal of Psychiatry*. The journal *Evidence-Based Mental Health* (EBMH) gives a summary of a selection of the best studies from over 50 leading international medical journals. In *EBMH* the key details of each chosen study are presented in an informative abstract with an additional expert commentary on its clinical application. Since *EBMH* is published quarterly, candidates are advised to go through the abstracts from the last eight issues before their examination.

One of the keys to examination success is to practise MCQs in the subject areas that regularly appear in the examination. We have covered all such areas in this book and provide a list of books useful in revision as well as the essential reference textbooks. We have used these books for reference in writing this MCQ book.

The best way to practise MCQs is in a group of candidates for the examination. In small groups, the recommended practice method is to solve MCQs by reading around the topic, and then comparing the answers and explanations given in the book. It is important to remember that this book is not a substitute for standard textbooks and should be used as a guide to focus on important examination topics. In this book we have not included page numbers of textbooks within the answers. Candidates are expected to read about the topics covered in the MCQ stem from the further reading references detailed at the end of the answer section in each chapter.

In the later part of revision, a few weeks before the examination, this book should be used as a practice examination, and 18 questions from each chapter should be solved in 2 hours (altogether 126 questions in one sitting), since the actual examination is 3 hours long and two-thirds of it consists of MCQs. Choosing different sets of multiples of 18 each time (for example, question numbers 1–18 from each chapter for the first practice examination and 19–36 for the second) will give the trainee the opportunity to undertake at least two practice examinations before the actual examination. Good time management is an important contributor to success and strict time keeping is essential in preparation for the examination.

It is also important to read and understand each stem thoroughly since some common terms used in MCQs may guide you to the correct response. Although there is no strict rule that any term indicates that the statement is true or false, the use of terms such as 'may', 'may be', 'can occur', 'can be', etc., could indicate an increased chance of the statement being true. Similarly, terms such as 'always occur' and 'never occur' could indicate the possibility of the statement being false.

Other terms such as 'characteristic', 'pathognomonic', 'common' and 'rare' should also be interpreted cautiously. Generally, 'characteristic' means that without the presence of that feature the diagnosis is doubtful; a 'pathognomonic' feature is found only in that condition; 'common' generally means found in more than 30%; and 'rare' means found in less than 5%.

We recommend working through the chapters of this book as early as possible before the examination date, reading around the topics given in a question stem from the books provided in the reading list and making notes for reference a few weeks before the examination. We suggest that you attempt the questions before checking the answers and any questions answered incorrectly should be noted and revised carefully in the weeks just before the examination. In this way we hope this book will be useful for consolidating your knowledge and helping you to get through the MRCPsych Paper 3 examination.

Arunraj Kaimal
Manoj Rajagopal
Salman Karim

Recommended reading

Preparation for the Paper 3 exam

British National Formulary. *BNF 57*. London: Pharmaceutical Press. Also available at: www.bnf.org/bnf.

Buckley P, Prewette D, Bird J, Harrison G. *Examination Notes in Psychiatry*, 4th edn. London: Hodder Education, 2004.

Gelder M, Harrison P, Cowen P. *Shorter Oxford Textbook of Psychiatry*, 5th edn. Oxford: Oxford University Press, 2006.

Hodges JR. *Cognitive Assessment for Clinicians*, 2nd edn. Oxford: Oxford University Press, 2007.

ICD-10: *The ICD-10 Classification of Mental and Behavioural Disorders: Clinical Descriptions and Diagnostic Guidelines*. Geneva: World Health Organization, 1990.

Munafo M. *Psychology for the MRCPsych*, 2nd edn. London: Hodder Education, 2002.

Oyebode F. *Sims' Symptoms in the Mind: An Introduction to Descriptive Psychopathology*, 4th edn. London: Saunders, 2008.

Puri B, Hall A. *Revision Notes in Psychiatry*, 2nd edn. London: Arnold/ Hodder Education, 2004.

Sadock BJ, Sadock VA. *Kaplan and Sadock's Synopsis of Psychiatry*, 10th edn. Baltimore, MD: Lippincott Williams and Wilkins, 2008.

Smith EE, Bem DJ, Nolen-Hoeksema S. Chapters 2–6. In: *Atkinson and Hilgard's Introduction to Psychology*, 14th edn. Florence, KY: Wadsworth Publishing Company, 2003.

Taylor D, Paton C, Kerwin R. *Maudsley Prescribing Guidelines*, 9th edn. London: Informa Healthcare, 2007.

Wright P, Stern J, Phelan M. *Core Psychiatry*, 2nd edn. London: Saunders, 2005.

General revision

David A, Fleminger S, Kopelman M, Lovestone S, Mellers J. *Lishman's Organic Psychiatry: A Textbook of Neuropsychiatry*, 4th edn. Chichester: Wiley-Blackwell, 2009.

Fish FJ, Casey PR, Kelly B. *Fish's Clinical Psychopathology: Signs and Symptoms in Psychiatry*, 3rd edn. London: Royal College of Psychiatrists Publications, 2007.

Gross R. *Psychology: The Science of Mind and Behaviour*, 5th edn. London: Hodder Education, 2005.

Kumar P, Clark M. *Kumar and Clark's Clinical Medicine*, 7th edn. London: Saunders, 2009.

Stahl SM. *Stahl's Essential Psychopharmacology: Neuroscientific Basis and Practical Applications*, 3rd edn. Cambridge: Cambridge University Press, 2008.

1) Regarding testamentary capacity, which of the following statements is correct?

   a. The term testamentary capacity is the same as fitness to plead
   b. If someone is suffering from a mental illness at the time of making a will, the will is not legally valid
   c. To decide that the testator is of sound disposing mind, he or she should know the exact nature and extent of the property, down to the smallest detail
   d. To decide that the testator is of sound disposing mind, he or she should know the names of close relatives and should be able to assess their claims to the property
   e. To decide that the testator is of sound disposing mind, he or she should be free from delusional thoughts

2) An 82-year-old woman admitted to the medical ward after being found unwell at her home by a carer complains to family members visiting her on the ward next day that the staff on the ward are stealing her things and poisoning her food. She appears bemused and bewildered and tells the family that there were hooded men around her bed the previous evening. The most probable diagnosis is:

   a. Schizophrenia
   b. Dementia
   c. Delusional disorder
   d. Drug-induced psychosis
   e. Delirium

3) A 48-year-old homeless man is brought to the A&E department in an agitated and confused state by paramedics. He complains of wavering vision and sees double when looking to the side. He needs support on walking and has a disturbed gait. On examination he has nystagmus and conjugate gait paralysis. An MRI scan performed using T2-dependent sequences shows abnormal high-intensity areas surrounding the third ventricles in the massa intermedia, the floor of the third ventricle, the mammillary bodies, the reticular formation and the periaqueductal region. The most appropriate treatment is:

   a. Intravenous acetylcysteine
   b. Intravenous naloxone
   c. Intravenous thiamine
   d. Intravenous glucose
   e. Intravenous flumazenil

4) A 44-year-old man is brought to the A&E department with disinhibition, ataxia and visual disturbances. On CT scan, hypodense areas are visible in the putamen; a T2-weighted MRI study shows high-intensity necrotic areas in the putamen. The most likely diagnosis is:

a. Systemic lupus erythematosus
b. Marchiafava–Bignami disease
c. Fahr syndrome
d. Carbon dioxide poisoning
e. Methanol intoxication

5) Immediately after a myocardial infarction, a 58-year-old man develops depression of moderate severity and has some deliberate self-harm ideations, but with no suicidal intentions; the preferred antidepressant of choice is:

a. Fluoxetine
b. Paroxetine
c. Sertraline
d. Duloxetine
e. Lofepramine

6) A 42-year-old woman is referred to you with a history of eating excessively and inappropriately after developing herpes encephalitis. There have been some changes in her personality, including increased agitation, and she has gained 12 kg in the last three months. Which of the following explains this presentation?

a. Prader–Willi syndrome
b. Klüver–Bucy syndrome
c. Kleine–Levin syndrome
d. Klinefelter syndrome
e. Kearns–Sayre syndrome

7) Sexual dysfunction associated with SSRIs is mediated mainly by:

a. 5-HT_1, etc. receptor stimulation
b. 5-HT_1, etc. receptor blockade
c. 5-HT_2, etc. receptor stimulation
d. 5-HT_2, etc. receptor blockade
e. 5-HT_3, etc. stimulation

8) NO-synthase inhibition by which of the following SSRIs may contribute to erectile dysfunction?

a. Fluoxetine
b. Paroxetine
c. Citalopram
d. Sertraline
e. Escitalopram

9) Which of the following antipsychotic drugs was shown to be useful in the prophylaxis of delirium?

a. Risperidone
b. Olanzapine
c. Haloperidol
d. Quetiapine
e. Aripiprazole

10) Regarding sexual dysfunction, all of the following statements are true, except:

a. Sexual dysfunction in the general population is more prevalent in men
b. Comparative studies indicate higher levels of sexual dysfunction in patients with depression than in controls
c. Comparative studies of SSRIs have generally found no significant differences between drugs in causing sexual dysfunction
d. Maprotiline and moclobemide are less likely to cause sexual dysfunction than amitriptyline and doxepin, respectively
e. Bupropion and nefazodone are less likely to cause sexual dysfunction than sertraline

11) In which of the following is the pulvinar sign seen on MRI?

a. Gerstmann–Sträussler–Scheinker syndrome
b. Huntington's chorea
c. Variant Creutzfeldt–Jakob disease
d. Lewy body dementia
e. Normal-pressure hydrocephalus

12) A 28-year-old man is brought to the A&E department complaining of acute onset of confusion. His relatives report that he has complained of a strange smell that others cannot perceive and has said that there is something churning in his stomach and rising towards his throat. He expresses an intense sense of familiarity with you and your surroundings. He also has flushing and tachycardia. The most probable diagnosis is:

a. Opioid withdrawal state
b. Schizoprenia
c. Complex partial seizure
d. Somatoform autonomic dysfunction
e. Conversion disorder

13) You have seen as an outpatient a 22-year-old man with progressive memory impairment and long-standing extrapyramidal symptoms, including rigidity, dystonia and choreoathetoid movements. His MRI scan was reported to have shown generalized brain atrophy and 'tiger's eye' appearance. The most probable diagnosis is:

a. Huntington's chorea
b. Fahr syndrome
c. Hallervorden–Spatz syndrome
d. Neuroacanthocytosis
e. Metachromatic leukodystrophy

14) ICD-10 confirms the diagnosis of enduring personality change after a catastrophic experience if the change has lasted for at least:

a. 6 months
b. 1 year
c. 2 years
d. 3 years
e. 4 years

15) Regarding biological abnormalities in people with personality disorders, all of the following statements are true, except:

a. Reduced prefrontal grey matter was observed in people with antisocial personality disorder
b. Deficits in the amygdala response to emotional stimuli were observed in people with antisocial personality disorder
c. A decreased volume of amygdala was observed in people with socio-pathic personalities
d. Increased levels of 5-hydroxyindoleacetic acid have been found in the cerebrospinal fluid of people who have committed unpremeditated violence
e. 5HT-mediated prolactin release is lower in subjects with histories of impulsive aggressiveness

16) Contraindications of zopiclone include all of the following, except:

a. Pregnancy
b. Unstable myasthenia gravis
c. Respiratory failure
d. Severe sleep apnoea
e. Breast feeding

17) Bilateral concentric visual field defects have been reported in patients treated with:

a. Lamotrigine
b. Sodium valproate
c. Gabapentin
d. Vigabatrin
e. Carbamazepine

18) A 40-year-old farmer referred by his GP to your outpatient department presents with a history of fatigue and low motivation for the last few weeks as well as arthritic pain on multiple joints. He appears low in mood and tells you that he has a rash on his chest, which is extending slowly. The most probable diagnosis is:

a. Chronic fatigue syndrome
b. Lyme disease
c. Fibromyalgia
d. Somatization disorder
e. Factitious disorder

19) All of the following statements regarding chronic fatigue syndrome are true, except:

a. Estimate of prevalence is between 0.3% and 1.5% of the general population
b. The diagnosis requires that the illness must have lasted for at least 6 months
c. Subjective memory impairment occurs
d. It is associated with tender lymph nodes
e. SSRIs are the treatment of choice, with proven efficacy

20) All of the following statements regarding fibromyalgia are true, except:

a. It is often accompanied by poor sleep, muscle aching and tenderness at trigger points
b. The arms and legs are affected more than other parts of the body
c. It is more common in women
d. It is more common in middle age
e. Controlled trials have shown the value of antidepressants

21) Regarding somatic symptoms unexplained by somatic pathology, which of the following statements is true?

a. When the diagnosis of factitious disorder, including the findings and their implications, is explained to patients, some admit that the symptoms are self-inflicted
b. The majority of people with irritable bowel syndrome consult a doctor
c. People with Munchausen syndrome usually encourage health professionals to obtain information about their previous treatments from other hospitals
d. In factitious disorder by proxy, gastrointestinal signs are most commonly reported
e. Malingering is not usually for the purpose of obtaining any gain

22) Which of the following statements about factitious disorder by proxy is true?

   a. Some children collude in the production of symptoms and signs
   b. Perpetrators usually have severe personality disorders and some may have a factitious disorder
   c. The prognosis is poor for children
   d. The prognosis is poor for perpetrators
   e. All of the above

23) A 34-year-old woman recently diagnosed with multiple sclerosis is developing increasingly severe depressive symptoms after starting treatment. The most probable pharmacological reason for this is treatment with:

   a. Beta interferon
   b. Cyclosporine
   c. Azathioprine
   d. Methotrexate
   e. Natalizumab

24) People with emotionally unstable personality disorder (borderline type) are believed to be operating in:

   a. Freud's anal stage of development
   b. Mahler's autistic stage
   c. Winnicott's false self
   d. Klein's paranoid-schizoid position
   e. Adler's inferiority complex

25) You are asked to assess a 24-year-old man who has been brought to your unit by the police. The police report that he has been involved in several violent crimes. In front of you he appears calm and knowledgeable about psychiatric problems and tells you that the police officers did not do their job properly as they did not arrest the people he was fighting with. When the police officer tries to interrupt him he suddenly becomes violent and kicks the officer. You have a discussion with his mother over the phone and she tells you that her son has had conduct disorder in the past and has low tolerance to frustration and a low threshold for aggression and violence. The most probable diagnosis is:

   a. Histrionic personality disorder
   b. Borderline personality disorder
   c. Attention deficit hyperactivity disorder
   d. Antisocial personality disorder
   e. Narcissistic personality disorder

26) Diagnostic criteria for borderline personality disorder include all of the following, except:

    a. Disturbance in and uncertainty about self-image, aims and internal preferences (including sexual)

    b. Liability to become involved in intense and unstable relationships, often leading to emotional crisis

    c. Excessive efforts to avoid abandonment

    d. Recurrent threats or acts of self-harm

    e. Chronic feeling of low mood and depression

27) Which of the following is least recommended in the management of antisocial personality disorder?

    a. Problem-solving counselling to help the patient deal with stressful circumstances that provoke abnormal behaviour or painful feelings

    b. Psychodynamic counselling to help the patient deal with stressful circumstances that provoke abnormal behaviour or painful feelings

    c. Antipsychotic drugs to calm the aggressive behaviour arising in response to increased stress

    d. Antidepressant medications to control the depressive symptoms associated with increased stress

    e. Anxiolytic drugs to control the mood and anxiety symptoms associated with increased stress

28) Obsessive compulsive disorder can be associated with:

    a. Gilles de la Tourette syndrome

    b. HIV infection

    c. Sydenham's chorea

    d. Multiple sclerosis

    e. All of the above

29) In severe obsessive compulsive disorder with obsessional rituals, the most appropriate treatment is:

    a. Clomipramine

    b. Exposure and response prevention

    c. Dynamic psychotherapy with SSRIs

    d. Neurosurgery

    e. Exposure and response prevention with SSRIs

30) All of the following statements about social phobia are true, except:

    a. Patients are often preoccupied with the idea of being observed critically

    b. It is a predictor of alcohol misuse

    c. Suicide attempts are more frequent than in the general population

    d. Positron emission tomography (PET) study of social phobics experiencing anticipatory anxiety found decreased blood flow in the right dorsolateral prefrontal cortex

    e. Successful treatment with citalopram or cognitive behavioural therapy results in decreased blood flow in the amygdala and related brain areas

31) Which of the following is the psychological treatment of choice for social phobia?

   a. Exposure and response prevention
   b. Relaxation training
   c. Supportive psychotherapy
   d. Cognitive behavioural therapy
   e. Dynamic psychotherapy

32) All of the following statements regarding generalized anxiety disorder (GAD) are true, except:

   a. Social phobia is the most common comorbid anxiety disorder occurring with GAD
   b. DSM-IV allows the diagnosis of mixed anxiety and depressive disorder
   c. Phaeochromocytoma and hypoglycaemia should be considered in the differential diagnosis of GAD
   d. Lifetime prevalence of GAD is around 5%, with women affected more than men
   e. Anxiety disorders lasting for more than 6 months have a poor prognosis

33) All of the following statements are true regarding primary depersonalization disorder, except:

   a. It is classified as a dissociative disorder in DSM-IV
   b. It is characteristically experienced as an unpleasant state by the patient
   c. It is possibly associated with schizoid personality disorder
   d. It is associated with a greater response in the insula and occipitotemporal cortex in an fMRI study
   e. In the majority of people depersonalization does not persist for a long time

34) In DSM-IV, the diagnosis of acute stress disorder requires: marked symptoms of anxiety or increased arousal; re-experiencing of the distressing event; and three dissociative symptoms from a list of five. All of the following are included in those dissociative symptoms, except:

   a. A sense of numbing or detachment
   b. Increased awareness of the surroundings
   c. Derealization
   d. Depersonalization
   e. Dissociative amnesia

35) All of the following are individual factors that increase vulnerability to the development of post-traumatic stress disorder, except:

   a. Previous history of trauma
   b. Female gender
   c. Neuroticism
   d. Higher intelligence
   e. Lack of social support

36) Which of the following is a neurobiological abnormality in post-traumatic stress disorder?

a. Low plasma cortisol level
b. Increased sensitivity to dexamethasone suppression
c. Increased levels of corticotropin-releasing hormone in the cerebrospinal fluid
d. Dysregulation of the hypothalamic–pituitary–adrenal axis
e. All of the above

37) Regarding the involvement of the monoamine neurotransmitter noradrenaline in the neurobiology of post-traumatic stress disorder (PTSD), all of the following statements are true, except:

a. Sympathetic tone is increased in PTSD
b. Startle response is increased in PTSD
c. MHPG level is decreased in the cerebrospinal fluid
d. There is an increased anxiety response to noradrenaline challenge
e. There is increased activity in noradrenergic innervation of the amygdala

38) A 40-year-old man presents as an outpatient with a history of anxiety, some insomnia and poor concentration after a car accident 3 weeks previously. He has had flashbacks and a few distressing dreams relating to the accident. The most appropriate management option is:

a. A critical incident debriefing (CID) and discharge back to the GP for primary-care follow-up
b. Watchful waiting and a follow-up appointment within a month
c. Short-term anxiolytic medication and urgent referral for trauma-focused cognitive behavioural treatment
d. Eye movement and desensitization reprocessing therapy
e. Citalopram to be started on 10 mg/day, with a view to increasing it in 3 weeks' time to 20 mg if there are no side-effects, and a follow-up appointment in 6 weeks

39) A 44-year-old man who lives with his wife comes to your outpatient clinic. He has appeared low in mood for the past 9 months since his mother's sudden and unexpected death. He wakes up early in the morning and sometimes hears his mother's voice calling him. Although he has had some thoughts about joining his mother in heaven he does not want to end his life. His wife says that he drinks a few days a week to get rid of the difficult thoughts from his head. In your assessment he meets the criteria for a depressive disorder of moderate severity. The most appropriate management plan is:

a. Admission to the inpatient ward and treatment with antipsychotic medication
b. Treatment with antidepressant medication
c. Grief counselling
d. Guided mourning
e. Cognitive behavioural therapy

40) All of the following statements about atypical depression are true, except:

a. Variably depressed mood with mood reactivity to positive events occurs
b. Symptoms include overeating and oversleeping
c. Extreme fatigue and heaviness in the limbs are features
d. Pronounced anxiety occurs
e. There is a better response to tricyclic antidepressants than to MAOIs and SSRIs

41) All of the following statements are true about rapid cycling disorder, except:

a. There should be at least four episodes a year separated by a period of remission or a switch to an episode of opposite polarity
b. It occurs more frequently in women
c. It can be triggered by antidepressant treatment
d. Concomitant hypothyroidism is common
e. Lithium is the most effective treatment as a mood stabilizer

42) Which of the following statements is true regarding seasonal affective disorder?

a. Onset occurs in autumn or winter and recovery in spring or summer
b. Symptoms include hypersomnia
c. Increased appetite with a craving for carbohydrate occurs
d. An afternoon slump in energy is a feature
e. All of the above

43) All of the following statements about mood disorders are true, except:

a. The point prevalence of depression is greater than that of bipolar illness
b. The mean age of onset is 10 years later in depression than in bipolar illness
c. The prevalence of depression and bipolar illness is twice as great in women as men
d. The risk of mood disorders is about twice as great in first-degree relatives of bipolar patients
e. It has been estimated that 10% of patients presenting with a depressive disorder will eventually have a manic illness

44) Abnormalities in monoamine neurotransmission in depression include all of the following, except:

  a. Increased plasma tryptophan
  b. Blunted 5-HT neuroendocrine responses
  c. Decreased brain 5-HT_{1A} receptor binding
  d. Decreased brain 5-HT reuptake sites
  e. Clinical relapse after tryptophan depletion

45) Regarding neurochemical abnormalities of depression, all of the following statements are true, except:

  a. Drug-free patients with major depression have a consistent reduction in cerebrospinal fluid (CSF) concentrations of 5-hydroxyindoleacetic acid (5-HIAA)
  b. Blunted noradrenaline-mediated growth hormone release is seen in depression
  c. Clinical relapse of depression occurs after administration of AMPT
  d. Decreased homovanillic acid (HVA) levels in the cerebrospinal fluid is seen in depression
  e. Increased dopamine D2 receptor binding occurs in depression

46) Low CSF 5-HIAA levels in patients who have made impulsive and more dangerous suicide attempts are observed in:

  a. Depression
  b. Schizophrenia
  c. Borderline personality disorder
  d. Antisocial personality disorder
  e. All of the above

47) About half of patients suffer from depression in which of the following?

  a. Cushing syndrome
  b. Addison's disease
  c. Hypothyroidism
  d. Hyperparathyroidism
  e. Hyperthyroidism

48) Blunted thyrotropin-stimulating hormone (TSH) response to intravenous thyrotropin-releasing hormone (TRH) is seen in all the following conditions, except:

  a. Depression
  b. Alcoholism
  c. Panic disorder
  d. Schizophrenia
  e. None of the above

49) Immune changes in depression include which of the following?

a. Lowered proliferative responses of lymphocytes to mitogens
b. Lowered natural killer cell activity
c. Increased positive acute phase proteins
d. Increased cytokine levels
e. All of the above

50) Sleep changes in depression include which of the following?

a. Impaired sleep continuity and duration
b. Decreased sleep stages 3 and 4
c. Decreased REM sleep latency
d. Increase in the proportion of REM sleep in the early part of the night
e. All of the above

1) d.
The term 'testamentary capacity' is the capacity to make a valid will. If a person has a mental illness at the time of making a will, its validity may be in doubt and it could be challenged. But the will is still legally valid if the testator is of sound disposing mind. To make sure that the testator is of sound disposing mind, he or she should know what the will is and its consequences, the nature and extent of the property (not necessarily in detail), and the names of close relatives, and he or she should be able to assess their claims to the property. The testator should not have an abnormal state of mind with distorted judgements affecting capability to make the will. A deluded person can make a valid will if that delusion does not distort his or her feelings or judgements relevant to making the will.

Gelder M, Harrison P, Cowen P. Chapter 4. In: *Shorter Oxford Textbook of Psychiatry*, 5th edn. Oxford: Oxford University Press, 2006.

2) e.
Typically the onset of delirium is acute and present in 18% of patients admitted to a geriatric ward and it increases to 24% in the course of their stay. Because of the acute onset, the patient is often perplexed and suspicious, with delusions and visual hallucinations.

Butler R, Pitt B. Chapter 3. In: *Seminars in Old Age Psychiatry*. London: Gaskell, 1998.

3) c.
The diagnosis is Wernicke's encephalopathy, with the characteristic clinical triad of confusion, ataxia and ophthalmoplegia, and radiological findings.

Lishman WA. Chapter 12. In: *Organic Psychiatry: The Psychological Consequences of Cerebral Disorder*, 3rd edn. Oxford: Wiley/Blackwell, 1997.
Scarabino T, Salvolini U, Jinkins RJ. *Emergency Neuroradiology*. New York: Springer, 2005.

4) e.
The initial presentation of methanol intoxication is the same as ethanol toxicity. Patients may develop headache, nausea, vomiting or epigastric pain and rapidly progress to obtundation and coma. Oculotoxicity may lead to blindness; neuroimaging reveals characteristic lesions in the putamen as described.

Scarabino T, Salvolini U, Jinkins RJ. *Emergency Neuroradiology*. New York: Springer, 2005.

5) c.

Fluoxetine, paroxetine and citalopram cause a small decrease in heart rate. Lofepramine increases heart rate moderately. With fluoxetine, paroxetine and lofepramine some cases of arrhythmias have been reported (Taylor *et al.* 2007). Meta-analysis of controlled trials of SSRIs has found no significant increases in suicidal ideation or suicidal acts, as compared with placebo or tricyclic antidepressants (Butler & Pitt 1998).

Butler R, Pitt B. Chapter 21. In: *Seminars in Old Age Psychiatry*. London: Gaskell, 1998.

Taylor D, Paton C, Kerwin R. *Maudsley Prescribing Guidelines*, 9th edn. London: Informa Healthcare, 2007.

6) b.

Klüver–Bucy syndrome is associated with temporal lobe abnormality. Kleine–Levin syndrome is associated with periodic somnolence and hyperphagia. In both syndromes hypersexuality can occur. Kearns–Sayre syndrome is mitochondrial myopathy.

Lishman WA. *Organic Psychiatry: The Psychological Consequences of Cerebral Disorder*, 3rd edn. Oxford: Wiley/Blackwell, 1997.

7) c.

By binding to serotonin, transporter SSRIs block the reuptake of released 5-HT and increase the concentration of 5-HT at its receptors, which are both post- and presynaptic. The 5-HT_1 receptor mediates antidepressant and anxiolytic activity and 5-HT_2 receptor stimulation mediates insomnia, agitation and sexual dysfunction. 5-HT_3 is associated with nausea and headaches.

Taylor D, Paton C, Kerwin R. Chapter 25. In: *Maudsley Prescribing Guidelines*, 9th edn. London: Informa Healthcare, 2007.

8) b.

Paroxetine, sertraline and citalopram have anticholinergic side-effects; the prolactin level is slightly raised by paroxetine and citalopram but not sertraline.

Taylor D, Paton C, Kerwin R. Chapter 25. In: *Maudsley Prescribing Guidelines*, 9th edn. London: Informa Healthcare, 2007.

9) c.

Kalisvaart *et al.* (2005) showed in a randomized placebo-controlled study that low-dose haloperidol prophylactic treatment demonstrated no efficacy in reducing the incidence of postoperative delirium. It did have a positive effect on the severity and duration of delirium. Moreover, haloperidol reduced the number of days patients stayed in the hospital, and the therapy was well tolerated (*British National Formulary 57*).

British National Formulary. *BNF 57*. London: Pharmaceutical Press. Also available at: www.bnf.org/bnf.

Kalisvaart KJ, de Jonghe JF, Bogaards MJ, *et al*. Haloperidol prophylaxis for elderly hip-surgery patients at risk for delirium: a randomized placebo-controlled study. *J Am Geriatr Soc* 2005; **53**: 1658–66.

10) a.
Sexual dysfunction in the general population is more prevalent in women (43%) than men (31%). There are probable advantages: of maprotiline and moclobemide over amitriptyline and doxepin, respectively; of bupropion (amfebutamone) and reboxetine over fluvoxamine; and of bupropion and nefazodone over sertraline.

Baldwin D, Mayers A. Sexual side-effects of antidepressant and antipsychotic drugs. *Adv Psychiatr Treat* 2003; **9**: 202–10.
Edwards JG. Newer *v*. older antidepressants in long-term pharmacotherapy. *Adv Psychiatr Treat* 2005; **11**: 184–94.

11) c.
The pulvinar sign on MRI is hyperintensity over the posterior thalamus (a useful and non-invasive diagnostic sign).

Gelder M, Harrison P, Cowen P. Chapter 14. In: *Shorter Oxford Textbook of Psychiatry*, 5th edn. Oxford: Oxford University Press, 2006.

12) c.
Complex partial seizure (temporal lobe epilepsy) presents with epigastric aura, autonomic signs and distorted perceptions, including olfactory hallucinations and déjà vu phenomena.

Gelder M, Harrison P, Cowen P. Chapter 14. In: *Shorter Oxford Textbook of Psychiatry*, 5th edn. Oxford: Oxford University Press, 2006.

13) c.
Hallervorden–Spatz syndrome is autosomal recessive and MRI shows destruction of the central part of the globus pallidus, surrounded by dark signal due to iron deposition ('tiger's eye' appearance).

Lishman WA. Chapter 15. In: *Organic Psychiatry: The Psychological Consequences of Cerebral Disorder*, 3rd edn. Oxford: Wiley/Blackwell, 1997.

14) c.
ICD-10 has three categories of change in personality: (1) due to organic disease of the brain classified in section F00; (2) enduring personality change after psychiatric illness; and (3) enduring personality change after a catastrophic experience. (2) and (3) are classified in section F60 and need the change to have lasted for at least 2 years.

Gelder M, Harrison P, Cowen P. Chapter 7. In: *Shorter Oxford Textbook of Psychiatry*, 5th edn. Oxford: Oxford University Press, 2006.

15) d.

Low levels of 5-hydroxyindoleacetic acid have been found in the cerebrospinal fluid of people who have committed unpremeditated violence.

Gelder M, Harrison P, Cowen P. Chapter 7. In: *Shorter Oxford Textbook of Psychiatry*, 5th edn. Oxford: Oxford University Press, 2006.

16) a.

As zopiclone can cause respiratory depression, muscle weakness and stable myasthenia gravis, caution is advised.

British National Formulary. *BNF 57*. London: Pharmaceutical Press. Also available at: www.bnf.org/bnf.

17) d.

The visual field defects associated with vigabatrin start from 1 month to several years after beginning treatment. In most cases the defects persist after discontinuation. Visual field testing before treatment is advised.

British National Formulary. *BNF 57*. London: Pharmaceutical Press. Also available at: www.bnf.org/bnf.

18) b.

Lyme disease is caused by the spirochaete *Borrelia burgdorferi*, which is transmitted to humans through tick bites. The tick bite is followed by the rash erythema migrans, a spreading annular erythema extending slowly outwards on the trunk or limbs, which is often a pointer to the diagnosis. Lyme disease is associated with neuropsychological problems and systemic disturbances.

Lishman WA. Chapter 8. In: *Organic Psychiatry: The Psychological Consequences of Cerebral Disorder*, 3rd edn. Oxford: Wiley/Blackwell, 1997.

19) e.

Many treatments have been suggested but very few are of proven efficacy. Cognitive behavioural therapy and graded exercise regimes have shown some benefits over standard medical care alone. When there is definite evidence of depressive disorder, antidepressants should be prescribed; SSRIs are better tolerated. Antidepressants are also useful in reducing anxiety, improving sleep and reducing pain.

Gelder M, Harrison P, Cowen P. Chapter 16. In: *Shorter Oxford Textbook of Psychiatry*, 5th edn. Oxford: Oxford University Press, 2006.

20) b.

The cervical and thoracic areas are affected most often but the pins may be located in the arms and legs. There is a marked association with depression and anxiety.

Gelder M, Harrison P, Cowen P. Chapter 16. In: *Shorter Oxford Textbook of Psychiatry*, 5th edn. Oxford: Oxford University Press, 2006.
Sadock BJ, Sadock VA. *Kaplan and Sadock's Synopsis of Psychiatry*, 10th edn. Baltimore, MD: Lippincott Williams and Wilkins, 2008.

21) a.

Irritable bowel syndrome occurs in as many as 10% of the general population, the majority of whom do not consult a doctor. People with Munchausen syndrome usually obstruct health professionals from obtaining information about their previous treatments from other hospitals. In factitious disorder by proxy, the signs reported most commonly are neurological, bleeding and rashes.

Gelder M, Harrison P, Cowen P. Chapter 16. In: *Shorter Oxford Textbook of Psychiatry*, 5th edn. Oxford: Oxford University Press, 2006.

22) e.

Hazards for children include disruption of education and social development. Occasional cases of murder are also reported.

Gelder M, Harrison P, Cowen P. Chapter 16. In: *Shorter Oxford Textbook of Psychiatry*, 5th edn. Oxford: Oxford University Press, 2006.

23) a.

Depression is a side-effect of beta interferon therapy and it is advised that it should not be used in people with severe depressive illness and suicidal ideation.

British National Formulary. *BNF 57*. London: Pharmaceutical Press. Also available at: www.bnf.org/bnf.
Gelder M, Harrison P, Cowen P. Chapter 14. In: *Shorter Oxford Textbook of Psychiatry*, 5th edn. Oxford: Oxford University Press, 2006.

24) d.

The paranoid-schizoid position is characterized by the predominance of primitive defence mechanisms, i.e. denial, splitting and primitive projective identification in the more mature depressive position. There is integration of good and bad aspects of self and others. Most people with borderline personalities operate more in the paranoid-schizoid than in the depressive position.

Wright P, Stern J, Phelan M. *Core Psychiatry*, 2nd edn. London: Saunders, 2005.

25) d.

Callous unconcern for the feelings of others, superficial charm, persistent disregard for social norms, low capacity for maintaining personal relationships, conduct disorder in childhood, low tolerance to frustration and low threshold for aggression and violence are all features of antisocial personality disorder.

Gelder M, Harrison P, Cowen P. Chapter 7. In: *Shorter Oxford Textbook of Psychiatry*, 5th edn. Oxford: Oxford University Press, 2006.
Puri B, Hall A. *Revision Notes in Psychiatry*, 2nd edn. London: Arnold/Hodder Education, 2004.

26) e.

ICD-10 requires a chronic feeling of emptiness (not low mood and depression).

ICD-10: The ICD-10 Classification of Mental and Behavioural Disorders: Clinical Descriptions and Diagnostic Guidelines. Geneva: World Health Organization, 1990.

27) e.

Anxiolytic drugs should be avoided as they may cause disinhibition and dependency.

Gelder M, Harrison P, Cowen P. Chapter 7. In: *Shorter Oxford Textbook of Psychiatry*, 5th edn. Oxford: Oxford University Press, 2006.

28) e.

Obsessive compulsive disorder is found in association with many organic brain diseases, including epilepsy and encephalitis lethargica.

Gelder M, Harrison P, Cowen P. *Shorter Oxford Textbook of Psychiatry*, 5th edn. Oxford: Oxford University Press, 2006.
Lishman WA. *Organic Psychiatry: The Psychological Consequences of Cerebral Disorder*, 3rd edn. Oxford: Wiley/Blackwell, 1997.
Sadock BJ, Sadock VA. *Kaplan and Sadock's Synopsis of Psychiatry*, 10th edn. Baltimore, MD: Lippincott Williams and Wilkins, 2008.

29) e.

Exposure and response prevention seem to produce better long-term results but it is difficult to achieve response prevention when symptoms are severe. For this reason, medication and response prevention should often be combined. Obsessional rituals usually respond very well to exposure and response prevention.

30) d.

A PET study of social phobics experiencing anticipatory anxiety found increased blood flow in the right dorsolateral prefrontal cortex, left inferior temporal cortex and left amygdaloid–hippocampal region.

Gelder M, Harrison P, Cowen P. Chapter 9. In: *Shorter Oxford Textbook of Psychiatry*, 5th edn. Oxford: Oxford University Press, 2006.

31) d.

A modified form of cognitive behavioural therapy based on particular cognitive abnormalities, coupled with measures to reduce safety behaviours, using video and audio feedback, was found to be more effective.

Gelder M, Harrison P, Cowen P. Chapter 9. In: *Shorter Oxford Textbook of Psychiatry*, 5th edn. Oxford: Oxford University Press, 2006.

32) b.

ICD-10 allows the diagnosis of mixed anxiety and depressive disorder, but in DSM-IV there is a need for both diagnoses if they occur together.

Gelder M, Harrison P, Cowen P. Chapter 9. In: *Shorter Oxford Textbook of Psychiatry*, 5th edn. Oxford: Oxford University Press, 2006.

33) d.

Primary depersonalization disorder is rare and is associated with a smaller response in the insula and occipitotemporal cortex in fMRI study and a greater response in the right ventral prefrontal cortex.

Gelder M, Harrison P, Cowen P. Chapter 10. In: *Shorter Oxford Textbook of Psychiatry*, 5th edn. Oxford: Oxford University Press, 2006.

34) b.

Reduced awareness of the surroundings and being in a daze is the dissociative symptom.

Gelder M, Harrison P, Cowen P. Chapter 8. In: *Shorter Oxford Textbook of Psychiatry*, 5th edn. Oxford: Oxford University Press, 2006.

35) d.

Factors summarized by Ozer *et al.* (2003) include lower intelligence and personal history of mood and anxiety disorder.

Gelder M, Harrison P, Cowen P. Chapter 8. In: *Shorter Oxford Textbook of Psychiatry*, 5th edn. Oxford: Oxford University Press, 2006.
Ozer EJ, Best SR, Lipsey TL, Weiss DS. Predictors of posttraumatic stress disorder and symptoms in adults: a meta-analysis. *Psychol Bull* 2003; **129**: 52–73.

36) e.

All these are found to be associated with abnormalities in the hypothalamic–pituitary–adrenal axis mediating defensive responses to stressful events, and there is a general increase in lability following environmental stress.

Gelder M, Harrison P, Cowen P. Chapter 8. In: *Shorter Oxford Textbook of Psychiatry*, 5th edn. Oxford: Oxford University Press, 2006.

37) c.

MHPG level is increased in the cerebrospinal fluid. The increased activity in noradrenergic innervation of the amygdala increases arousal and facilitates the automatic encoding and recall of traumatic memories.

38) b.

According to guidance from the National Institute for Health and Clinical Excellence (NICE) on the management of post-traumatic stress disorder and related traumatic syndromes, where symptoms are mild and have been present for less than 4 weeks after the trauma, watchful waiting and a follow-up appointment within a month are recommended.

Gelder M, Harrison P, Cowen P. Chapter 8, box on p. 162. In: *Shorter Oxford Textbook of Psychiatry*, 5th edn. Oxford: Oxford University Press, 2006.

39) b.

Antidepressants are beneficial if criteria for depressive disorders are met.

Gelder M, Harrison P, Cowen P. Chapter 8. In: *Shorter Oxford Textbook of Psychiatry*, 5th edn. Oxford: Oxford University Press, 2006.

40) e.

There is a better response to MAOIs and SSRIs and a poorer response to tricyclic antidepressants.

Gelder M, Harrison P, Cowen P. Chapter 11. In: *Shorter Oxford Textbook of Psychiatry*, 5th edn. Oxford: Oxford University Press, 2006.

41) e.

Lithium treatment is relatively ineffective.

Gelder M, Harrison P, Cowen P. Chapter 11. In: *Shorter Oxford Textbook of Psychiatry*, 5th edn. Oxford: Oxford University Press, 2006.

42) e.

It was suggested that shortening of daylight hours is important in pathophysiology; exposure to bright artificial light during hours of darkness is used as treatment.

Gelder M, Harrison P, Cowen P. Chapter 11. In: *Shorter Oxford Textbook of Psychiatry*, 5th edn. Oxford: Oxford University Press, 2006.

43) c.

The prevalence of bipolar illness in men and women is the same; the rates of major depression are about twice as great in women as in men; the lifetime risk of bipolar disorder is between 0.3% and 1.5%; the 5- and 6-month prevalence is not much less than the lifetime prevalence as the illness is chronic. Mean age of onset for bipolar illness is 17 and that of depression is 27 (Gelder *et al.* 2006); the point prevalence of depression is 1.8–3.2% in men and 2–9.3% in women, and that of bipolar illness is 0.6–1.1% (Puri & Hall 2004).

Gelder M, Harrison P, Cowen P. Chapter 11. In: *Shorter Oxford Textbook of Psychiatry*, 5th edn. Oxford: Oxford University Press, 2006.
Puri B, Hall A. *Revision Notes in Psychiatry*, 2nd edn. London: Arnold/ Hodder Education, 2004.

44) a.
Decreased plasma tryptophan occurs in depression. Tryptophan is the precursor of 5-HT.

Gelder M, Harrison P, Cowen P. Chapter 11. In: *Shorter Oxford Textbook of Psychiatry*, 5th edn. Oxford: Oxford University Press, 2006.

45) a.
Overall research evidence does not suggest that drug-free patients with major depression have a consistent reduction in cerebrospinal fluid (CSF) concentrations of 5-hydroxyindoleacetic acid (5-HIAA).

Gelder M, Harrison P, Cowen P. Chapter 11. In: *Shorter Oxford Textbook of Psychiatry*, 5th edn. Oxford: Oxford University Press, 2006.

46) e.
It has been proposed that low levels of CSF 5-HIAA, while not related specifically to depression, may be associated with a tendency for individuals to respond in an impulsive and hostile way to life difficulties.

Gelder M, Harrison P, Cowen P. Chapter 11. In: *Shorter Oxford Textbook of Psychiatry*, 5th edn. Oxford: Oxford University Press, 2006.

47) a.
In Cushing syndrome, depression usually remits when cortisol hypersecretion is corrected.

Gelder M, Harrison P, Cowen P. Chapter 11. In: *Shorter Oxford Textbook of Psychiatry*, 5th edn. Oxford: Oxford University Press, 2006.

48) d.
Normal thyrotropin-stimulating hormone (TSH) response to intravenous thyrotropin-releasing hormone (TRH) is observed in schizophrenia. It is also observed that in schizophrenia there is a blunted release of prolactin and growth hormone on thyroid-releasing hormone stimulation.

Gelder M, Harrison P, Cowen P. Chapter 11. In: *Shorter Oxford Textbook of Psychiatry*, 5th edn. Oxford: Oxford University Press, 2006.
Sadock BJ, Sadock VA. *Kaplan and Sadock's Synopsis of Psychiatry*, 10th edn. Baltimore, MD: Lippincott Williams and Wilkins, 2008.

49) e.

Cytokines are known to provoke hypothalamic–pituitary–adrenal (HPA) axis activity and therefore changes in immunoregulation may play a part in HPA axis dysfunction in depression.

Gelder M, Harrison P, Cowen P. Chapter 11. In: *Shorter Oxford Textbook of Psychiatry*, 5th edn. Oxford: Oxford University Press, 2006.

50) e.

Decreased REM sleep latency may persist in recovered depressed patients and indicate a vulnerability to relapse.

Gelder M, Harrison P, Cowen P. Chapter 11. In: *Shorter Oxford Textbook of Psychiatry*, 5th edn. Oxford: Oxford University Press, 2006.

Further reading

Baldwin D, Mayers A. Sexual side-effects of antidepressant and antipsychotic drugs. *Adv Psychiatr Treat* 2003; **9**: 202–10.

British National Formulary. *BNF 57*. London: Pharmaceutical Press. Also available at: www.bnf.org/bnf.

Butler R, Pitt B. *Seminars in Old Age Psychiatry*. London: Gaskell, 1998.

Edwards JG. Newer *v.* older antidepressants in long-term pharmacotherapy. *Adv Psychiatr Treat* 2005; **11**: 184–94.

Gelder M, Harrison P, Cowen P. *Shorter Oxford Textbook of Psychiatry*, 5th edn. Oxford: Oxford University Press, 2006.

ICD-10: The ICD-10 Classification of Mental and Behavioural Disorders: Clinical Descriptions and Diagnostic Guidelines. Geneva: World Health Organization, 1990.

Kalisvaart KJ, de Jonghe JF, Bogaards MJ, *et al*. Haloperidol prophylaxis for elderly hip-surgery patients at risk for delirium: a randomized placebo-controlled study. *J Am Geriatr Soc* 2005; **53**: 1658–66.

Lishman WA. *Organic Psychiatry: The Psychological Consequences of Cerebral Disorder*, 3rd edn. Oxford: Wiley/Blackwell, 1997.

Puri B, Hall A. *Revision Notes in Psychiatry*, 2nd edn. London: Arnold/ Hodder Education, 2004.

Sadock BJ, Sadock VA. *Kaplan and Sadock's Synopsis of Psychiatry*, 10th edn. Baltimore, MD: Lippincott Williams and Wilkins, 2008.

Scarabino T, Salvolini U, Jinkins RJ. *Emergency Neuroradiology*. New York: Springer, 2005.

Taylor D, Paton C, Kerwin R. *Maudsley Prescribing Guidelines*, 9th edn. London: Informa Healthcare, 2007.

Wright P, Stern J, Phelan M. *Core Psychiatry*, 2nd edn. London: Saunders, 2005.

1) Which of the following is a consistently observed neuroradiological finding in elderly people with late-onset depression?

   a. Enlarged lateral ventricles
   b. Decreased hippocampal volume
   c. Decreased volume of basal ganglia
   d. Frontotemporal cortex atrophy
   e. Decreased volume of amygdala

2) On MRI examination of the brain in depressive subjects, increased deep white matter hyperintensities are associated with:

   a. Late-onset depression
   b. Mild depression
   c. Good treatment response
   d. Psychomotor agitation
   e. Personality disorder

3) Neuropathological abnormalities observed in patients with mood disorders include which of the following?

   a. Increased synaptic markers in the prefrontal cortex
   b. Increased neuronal size in the prefrontal cortex
   c. Increased neuronal density in the prefrontal cortex
   d. Increased glial cell numbers in the cingulate cortex
   e. None of the above

4) In which of the following is there altered cerebral blood flow in patients with depression?

   a. Prefrontal cortex
   b. Anterior cingulate cortex
   c. Thalamus
   d. Caudate nucleus
   e. All of the above

5) Regarding lithium augmentation in depression, which of the following statements is true?

   a. According to research evidence it is more effective than placebo
   b. Most people respond with an amelioration of their depressive state within 24–48 hours after commencement of lithium
   c. Unipolar depressed patients do not respond so well as bipolar patients
   d. The dexamethasone suppression test is reliable in identifying patients likely to respond to lithium
   e. It is effective only when lithium is combined with SSRIs

6) There is no research evidence to support the claim that electro-convulsive therapy (ECT) is more effective than:

   a. Simulated ECT in major depression
   b. Tricyclic antidepressant treatment in major depression
   c. MAOI antidepressant treatment in major depression
   d. Antipsychotic treatment in depressive psychosis
   e. Combined tricyclic antidepressant and antipsychotic treatment in depressive psychosis

7) Regarding longer-term treatment for mood disorders, all of the following statements are true, except:

   a. Continuing antidepressants for 6 months after remission decreases the relapse rate by 50%
   b. Mood-incongruent psychotic features predict good response to lithium maintenance treatment
   c. Use of lithium maintenance treatment in recurrent mood disorders reduces suicide rates
   d. Carbamazepine is useful in prophylaxis of rapid cycling disorders
   e. Lamotrigine is effective in prophylaxis of bipolar depression

8) Common indications for treatment with SSRIs in depression include all of the following, except:

   a. Significant history of heart disease
   b. Concurrent treatment with anticholinergic drugs
   c. Risk of overdose
   d. Tendency to gain weight
   e. Sedation desirable

9) A 54-year-old woman is brought to the casualty department with acute onset of confusion and agitation. On examination she appears to be febrile, and has been sweating excessively. She is also found to have myoclonus and nystagmus. A careful history reveals that she has had chronic depression, hypertension and diabetes mellitus. She has been on insulin, phenelzine, atenolol and ramipril, and because of ongoing depressive symptoms clomipramine was added to her prescription recently. The most probable cause of her presentation is:

   a. Neuroleptic malignant syndrome
   b. Hypoglycaemia
   c. Serotonin syndrome
   d. Urinary tract infection
   e. Wernicke's encephalopathy

10) All of the following statements are true regarding velocardiofacial syndrome, except:

   a. It is also known as DiGeorge syndrome
   b. It is caused by deletion of one copy of chromosome 21
   c. It is associated with cognitive impairment
   d. 70% of cases are associated with psychosis
   e. It is a rare cause of schizophrenia

11) Regarding antipsychotic treatments for schizophrenia, all of the following statements are true, except:

   a. Drug treatment has more effect on positive symptoms than on negative symptoms
   b. Antipsychotics given at the first sign of relapse are more effective than continuous prophylaxis
   c. Depot medications are more effective in preventing relapse than oral medications
   d. There is some research evidence favouring the use of atypical antipsychotics rather than typical ones in the prophylaxis of schizophrenia
   e. The efficacy of clozapine is superior to that of other antipsychotics

12) All of the following statements are true regarding treatment with clozapine, except:

   a. Clozapine has proven efficacy in treatment-resistant schizophrenia
   b. Clozapine reduces mortality with suicide in schizophrenia
   c. Clozapine may be useful in the first episode of schizophrenia in treatment-naive patients as clear superiority is proven in comparison with chlorpromazine
   d. Antipsychotic polypharmacy may be justified in clozapine-resistant schizophrenia
   e. In clozapine-resistant schizophrenia, augmentation with lamotrigine and valproate may be useful

13) Regarding the management of acute episodes of schizophrenia, which of the following statements is not true?

   a. Hospital admission is usually indicated in the first episode
   b. A drug-free observation period may be helpful in the diagnosis
   c. Antipsychotic medication should be initiated soon after diagnosis
   d. In the acute phase, intramuscular medications are preferable to oral medications
   e. Anticholinergic drugs should not be given routinely to prevent extrapyramidal symptoms

14) Antipsychotic drugs are associated with all of the following, except:

    a. Increased risk of cerebrovascular events
    b. Insulin resistance
    c. Dyslipidaemia
    d. Osteoporosis
    e. Shortened QTc interval

15) Regarding the prognosis of schizophrenia, all of the following statements are true, except:

    a. Early treatment is associated with better prognosis
    b. Much of the deterioration in social functioning takes place later on in the illness, especially after 10 years
    c. Good premorbid functioning is a risk factor for suicide
    d. Patients with prolonged negative symptoms are less likely to attempt suicide
    e. Clozapine treatment significantly reduces suicide risk in schizophrenia

16) Regarding the prognosis of schizophrenia, all of the following statements are true, except:

    a. Treatment response time increases with increasing number of relapses
    b. According to an Epidemiologic Catchment Area (ECA) study in the USA, patients with schizophrenia have a four- to fivefold increased risk of substance abuse
    c. In half of violent schizophrenic patients, the violent behaviour can be directly attributed to psychotic symptoms like delusions
    d. Suicide risk is increased early in the course of the illness
    e. The mortality rate in women with schizophrenia is twice that in men

17) Regarding pathological jealousy, all of the following statements are true, except:

    a. Delusions of jealousy are more common in females with paranoid schizophrenia than in males with paranoid schizophrenia
    b. Delusions of jealousy are more common in males with alcoholic psychosis than in females with alcoholic psychosis
    c. The mainstay of treatment is antipsychotic drugs
    d. If there is a risk of violence, the doctor should warn a partner (even if that means breaching confidentiality)
    e. Patients usually respond very well to combined treatment with anti-psychotics and cognitive behavioural therapy

18) Regarding head injury, all of the following statements are true, except:

   a. The duration of post-traumatic amnesia (PTA) is a good indicator of the severity of a closed head injury
   b. PTA of less than 1 week indicates a better chance of returning to work
   c. Retrograde amnesia is a better predictor of outcome than PTA
   d. Deposition of beta amyloid may explain the link between head injury and Alzheimer's disease
   e. Apolipoprotein E4 genotype may increase the risk of death after head injury

19) All of the following statements regarding postconcussion syndrome are true, except:

   a. It is associated with anxiety and depression
   b. It is accompanied by headache and difficulties in concentration
   c. It occurs only after severe head injury
   d. It can be of psychological origin
   e. It mostly resolves without treatment

20) Regarding Gilles de la Tourette syndrome, all of the following statements are true, except:

   a. Multiple tics begin before the age of 16
   b. 30% of people with the syndrome have coprolalia
   c. Obsessive compulsive symptoms are seen
   d. Attention deficit hyperactivity disorder occurs frequently
   e. Antipsychotics are contraindicated

21) All of the following statements are true regarding multiple sclerosis, except:

   a. Psychological symptoms appear in two-thirds of patients
   b. Psychological symptoms are usually the presenting features
   c. It is associated with increased risk of suicide
   d. Rapidly progressive dementia may occur
   e. Cognitive impairment correlates with the degree of callosal atrophy

22) Which of the following statements is true regarding anorexia nervosa?

   a. Amenorrhoea precedes weight loss in 50% of patients
   b. Lack of sexual interest is usual
   c. High levels of T3 and T4 with low levels of thyroid-stimulating hormone (TSH) are a usual biochemical finding
   d. Decreased growth hormone concentration occurs
   e. 25% of patients eventually develop schizophrenia

23) Regarding the prognosis of anorexia nervosa, all of the following statements are true, except:

   a. It is associated with a sixfold increase in mortality
   b. The usual causes of death include suicide
   c. 20% of patients recover fully
   d. 20% of patients remain severely ill
   e. Onset at a younger age is a bad prognostic indicator

24) All of the following are abnormalities found in anorexia nervosa, except:

   a. Low concentrations of luteinizing hormone
   b. Increased plasma cortisol
   c. Dexamethasone non-suppression
   d. Hypercholesterolaemia
   e. Hyperkalaemia

25) Which of the following statements is true regarding restoration of weight in anorexia nervosa?

   a. It is usually done as an outpatient
   b. The aim is to increase body weight by 0.5 kg a week
   c. It requires an extra 500–1000 calories per day
   d. The usual target weight is between a healthy weight and a weight the patient thinks is ideal
   e. All of the above

26) Regarding the management of bulimia nervosa, all of the following statements are true, except:

   a. The most effective treatment is a special form of cognitive behavioural therapy (CBT)
   b. 30–50% of patients improve with therapy
   c. SSRIs do not appear to be beneficial as treatment
   d. A treatment combination of CBT and antidepressants does not have any advantage over treatment with CBT alone
   e. Interpersonal psychotherapy may be as effective as CBT, but takes longer to be effective

27) Which of the following statements is true regarding Kleine–Levin syndrome?

   a. It consists of episodes of sleep lasting for days or weeks with long periods of normality in between
   b. Increased appetite occurs
   c. Hypothalamic dysfunction is suggested in the aetiology
   d. Lithium may be useful in the treatment
   e. All of the above

28) Which of the following statements is true regarding sleepwalking disorder?

a. It is more common in children between 5 and 12 years of age
b. It may be familial
c. It occurs in approximately 15% of children
d. It rarely lasts as much as an hour
e. All of the above

29) All of the following statements are correct regarding suicide, except:

a. 30–50% of people who commit suicide are diagnosed with personality disorder
b. 10% of people with mood disorder die by suicide
c. There are higher rates in male doctors than female doctors
d. In most countries, the highest rate is reported in the population above 75 years old
e. Rates among adolescents have increased recently

30) Regarding psychiatric aspects of pregnancy, all of the following statements are true, except:

a. Psychiatric disorder is more common in the second trimester than in the first and third
b. Women with chronic psychological problems may improve during pregnancy
c. Eating disorders are not precipitated by pregnancy
d. Pseudocyesis is more common in younger women
e. In Couvade syndrome, the man complains of morning sickness

31) Which of the following statements is true regarding premenstrual syndrome?

a. It may present with a craving for food
b. There is decreased prevalence in those around 30 years of age
c. Lack of oestrogen and excess progesterone have been postulated as an aetiological mechanism
d. There is a low response rate to placebo
e. Bromocriptine is the only effective treatment

32) All of the following are associated with premenstrual syndrome, except:

a. High CNS beta endorphin levels
b. EEG changes
c. Alteration in response to dichotic auditory stimuli
d. Alterations in skin conductance
e. Type A behaviour

33) Which of the following is useful in treating premenstrual syndrome?

    a. SSRIs
    b. Oral contraceptive pill
    c. Vitamin B6
    d. Diuretics
    e. All of the above

34) All of the following are features of cyclic psychosis, except:

    a. Psychotic symptoms appearing suddenly before menstruation
    b. Tonic–clonic fits
    c. Transitory EEG abnormalities
    d. Psychomotor retardation
    e. Amnesia

35) The recommended treatment for cyclic psychosis includes:

    a. Bromocriptine
    b. Progesterone
    c. Clomiphene citrate
    d. Acetazolamide
    e. All of the above

36) Which of the following factors is associated with miscarriage?

    a. Severe life events in the 3 months before miscarriage
    b. Childhood maternal separation
    c. Poor relationship with partners
    d. Few social contacts
    e. All of the above

37) All of the following statements are true regarding postnatal blues, except:

    a. They occur in about 80% of mothers
    b. Peak incidence occurs between 3 and 5 days in the postpartum period
    c. They are associated with a history of premenstrual tension
    d. Serum calcium may play a role in their occurrence
    e. They are associated with a history of poor marital relationship

38) All of the following statements are true regarding postpartum depression, except:

    a. It occurs in 10–15% of mothers
    b. It usually occurs in the first 3 months postpartum
    c. There is an increased incidence in multiparous women
    d. Past psychiatric history is a risk factor
    e. The Edinburgh Postnatal Depression Scale is useful in identifying cases

39) All of the following statements are true regarding the management of postnatal depression, except:

a. Counselling by health visitors is effective
b. Self-help groups are useful
c. Antidepressants may be required
d. ECT is recommended in severe cases
e. Lithium is routinely given, as it has been proven effective

40) Which of the following statements is true regarding postnatal depression?

a. It may last for a few years
b. It can cause cognitive abnormalities in children of affected mothers
c. There is a raised risk for further episodes of postnatal depression
d. It is associated with an increased rate of thyroid dysfunction in the postpartum year
e. All of the above

41) All of the following are features of puerperal psychosis, except:

a. Onset is gradual, in the first few months after childbirth
b. It is not associated with cognitive impairment
c. The majority of cases are affective psychosis
d. It is more common in primiparae
e. There is an increased occurrence in higher social classes

42) All of the following statements are true regarding puerperal psychosis, except:

a. There is a higher risk in women with schizophrenia than in women with bipolar illness
b. Most patients recover fully
c. Most sufferers are capable of looking after their baby with support
d. Joint admission with the baby may reduce the duration of illness and relapse rate
e. ECT is often the best treatment in severe cases

43) In the assessment of sexual dysfunction, each partner should be asked:

a. Whether the problem has occurred with more than one partner
b. About masturbation
c. About frequency of intercourse
d. The sexual techniques of the other partner
e. All of the above

44) Which of the following statements is true regarding sex therapy?

    a. It involves education about the anatomy and physiology of intercourse
    b. It is not helpful in the majority of patients
    c. Better results are obtained if couples are treated separately
    d. A spectator role is encouraged in graded tasks
    e. If successful, the improvement is usually sustained for years

45) In a psychotherapeutic intervention, a patient tells you about her experience of her boss shouting at her because she arrived late at the office on one occasion. You say, 'It must have been really difficult for you. I can understand why you feel anxious about that.' This is an example of:

    a. Interpretation
    b. Affirmation
    c. Clarification
    d. Advice and praise
    e. Empathic validation

46) A depressed 44-year-old woman who has come for her first session of psychotherapy gets worked up because her husband is late in coming to the hospital to pick her up. She becomes tearful and tells the receptionist that she is worried that he has been involved in an accident. This is an example of:

    a. Interpretation
    b. Exaggeration
    c. Catastrophizing
    d. Overgeneralizing
    e. Ignoring the positive

47) All of the following are therapeutic factors in group therapy, except:

    a. Shared experience
    b. Formation of subgroups
    c. Group cohesion
    d. Interpersonal learning
    e. Recapitulation of the family group

48) The underlying principles of therapeutic community include:

    a. Democracy
    b. Reality confrontation
    c. Permissiveness
    d. Community
    e. All of the above

49) Bloch and Harari's framework for assessment of family function includes all of the following, except:

a. Family structure recorded in the genogram
b. Changes and events, including financial problems
c. Relationships (including conflicts)
d. Patterns of interaction involving two or more people in the family
e. Role of transference in shaping the interactions between family members

50) All of the following are true about *Hypericum perforatum*, except:

a. It is more effective than placebo in moderate depression
b. The most common side-effects include gastrointestinal disturbances
c. It may induce mania
d. It is a hepatic enzyme inducer
e. It is safe to use with SSRIs

51) The risk of Ebstein's anomaly associated with first-trimester use of lithium is:

a. 1/200 births
b. 1/2000 births
c. 1/20 000 births
d. 1/200 000 births
e. 1/100 000 births

52) The neural-tube defects in offspring associated with valproate use in the first trimester of pregnancy could be as high as:

a. 0.5%
b. 5%
c. 10%
d. 20%
e. 50%

53) Use of which of the following in pregnancy is associated with the highest risk of congenital malformation in children?

a. Lithium
b. Carbamazepine
c. Valproate
d. Lamotrigine
e. **b**, **c** and **d** carry equal risk

54) All of the following statements regarding atomoxetine are true, except:

   a. It is a noradrenaline reuptake inhibitor
   b. It is licensed for treatment of ADHD
   c. Sleep disturbance is a common side-effect
   d. Hepatic damage is a rare side-effect
   e. It is safe in angle-closure glaucoma

55) All of the following statements regarding Huntington's disease are true, except:

   a. Initial insight may result in depression
   b. Schizophrenia-like psychosis occurs
   c. Serpentine tongue is a typical feature
   d. There is an increased concentration of GABA in the caudate nucleus
   e. Gaze apraxia is found

56) Which of the following statements is true regarding Huntington's disease?

   a. The gene is located on chromosome 16
   b. The average time to death after diagnosis is 5 years
   c. It is associated with increased risk of suicide
   d. An increased volume of caudate is observed
   e. It causes rapidly progressing dementia

57) HIV dementia is associated with which of the following?

   a. Reduced libido early on
   b. Incontinence
   c. Ataxia
   d. Hyperreflexia
   e. All of the above

58) Which of the following statements is true regarding HIV infection?

   a. Associated dementia occurs in 50% of HIV-infected patients
   b. The most common infection is cytomegalovirus infection of the central nervous system
   c. Dementia is slowly progressing
   d. A progression from mild neurocognitive disorder to dementia cannot be prevented by antiviral treatment
   e. Depression is more common in men than in women

59) Protease inhibitors increase the concentration of all the following, except:

    a. SSRIs
    b. Aripiprazole
    c. Valproate
    d. Zolpidem
    e. Bupropion

60) Which of the following is a protease inhibitor?

    a. Zidovudine
    b. Zalcitabine
    c. Nevirapine
    d. Delavirdine
    e. Ritonavir

2. General adult psychiatry 2: Answers

1) a.
Decreased hippocampal volume and decreased volume of basal ganglia are observed in patients with unipolar depressive disorder. Decreased volume of grey matter in the subgenual prefrontal cortex is found in unipolar and bipolar illnesses. Increased volume of amigdala is seen in bipolar illness.

2) a.
Increased deep white matter hyperintensities are also associated with vascular risk factors, severe depression, poor treatment response and psychomotor retardation.

3) e.
All are decreased, not increased.

4) e.
Altered blood flow and metabolism are observed in all the regions in **a** to **d**, as well as amygdala.

5) a.
Amelioration of the depressive state can occur within 24–48 hours after commencement of lithium but usually symptoms resolve over 2–3 weeks; unipolar patients respond as well as bipolar patients; there are no reliable clinical or biochemical predictors; the effect is not restricted to any particular class of antidepressants.

6) e.
It has been observed that in depressive psychosis, combined tricyclic antidepressant and antipsychotic treatment may be as effective as ECT but there is no research evidence. There is research evidence for **a** to **d**.

The UK ECT Review Group. Electroconvulsive therapy: systematic review and meta-analysis of efficacy and safety in depressive disorders. *Lancet* 2003; **361**: 799–808.

7) b.
Mood-incongruent psychotic features predict poor response to lithium maintenance treatment.

8) e.
SSRIs are indicated for treatment of depression when sedation is undesirable.

9) c.

When serotoninergic drugs like clomipramine are combined with MAOIs like phenelzine, serotonin syndrome occurs, with the clinical features mentioned.

10) d.

30% of cases are associated with schizophrenia-like or affective psychosis.

11) b.

Continuous treatment is more effective than intermittent treatment.

12) c.

The superiority of clozapine in the first episode of schizophrenia in treatment-naive patients was not proven in a one-year trial.

Lieberman JA, Phillips M, Gu H, *et al.* Atypical and conventional antipsychotic drugs in treatment-naive first-episode schizophrenia: a 52-week randomized trial of clozapine vs chlorpromazine. *Neuropsychopharmacology* 2003; **28**: 995–1003.

13) d.

Oral medications are always preferable, but intramuscular medications may be necessary to control disturbed behaviour in patients who are not compliant with oral treatment.

14) e.

Antipsychotic drugs cause a prolonged QTc interval. Osteoporosis can result from hyperprolactinaemia.

15) b.

Much of the deterioration in social functioning takes place in the first 2 years after diagnosis.

16) e.

The mortality rate in men with schizophrenia is twice that in women.

17) e.

The general impression is that the prognosis is poor and only marginal benefits are reported with treatment.

18) c.

Retrograde amnesia has less predictive value.

19) c.

Postconcussion syndrome often occurs after mild head injury.

20) e.
Haloperidol and risperidone are an effective treatment; echolalia and echopraxia occur in 10–40%.

21) b.
Psychological symptoms are rarely the presenting features.

22) b.
Amenorrhoea precedes weight loss in 20% of patients; low levels of T3 and low normal T4 with normal TSH is a usual biochemical finding; raised growth hormone concentration is seen. Anorexia does not evolve into shizophrenia.

23) e.
Onset at a younger age is associated with better prognosis.

24) e.
Hypokalaemia occurs.

25) e.
Inpatient admission is indicated where there are life-threatening physical complications, severe depression and increased suicidal risk.

26) c.
SSRIs decrease the frequency of binge eating and purging and help in improving the mood.

27) e.
An autonomic basis is proposed.

28) e.
An episode of sleepwalking disorder usually lasts for only a few seconds or minutes, and rarely lasts up to an hour.

29) b.
6% of people with mood disorder die by suicide.

30) a.
Psychiatric disorder is more common in the first and third trimester than in the second trimester.

31) a.
There is increased prevalence in those around 30 years of age; lack of progesterone and excess oestrogen have been postulated as an aetiological mechanism; there is a high response rate to placebo; bromocriptine is used in treatment, but no drugs have been proven to be effective.

32) a.
Low CNS beta endorphin levels are associated with premenstrual syndrome.

33) e.
Bromocriptine and benzodiazepines are also used.

34) b.
EEG abnormalities not amounting to epilepsy can occur.

35) e.
Bromocriptine reduces prolactin and progesterone inhibits ovulation; psychotropic drugs are also used.

36) e.
Major social difficulty and severe short-term life event in the first 2 weeks immediately prior miscarriage are associated with miscarriage.

37) a.
Postnatal blues occur in half of mothers.

38) c.
It was not observed to be associated with parity.

39) e.
Lithium is not usually given, as it is secreted in the breast milk and is toxic to the child.

40) e.
Postpartum thyroid dysfunction peaks at 4–5 months.

41) a.
Onset is abrupt, in the first few weeks.

42) a.
Risk is higher in bipolar illness than in schizophrenia.

43) e.
Each partner should also be asked about sexual thoughts, feelings, social relationships, etc.

44) a.
Sex therapy is successful in 30% of cases and there is some improvement in a further 30%; better results are obtained if a couple are treated together; the 'spectator role' is checking their own arousal, which has an

inhibitory effect and should be discouraged; improvement is usually maintained for months and seldom for more than 3 years.

45) e.
Empathic validation helps patients to feel that the therapist understands their inner feelings and they are more likely to accept interpretations.

46) c.
It is one of the logical errors occurring in depressive disorders.

47) b.
Formation of subgroups disrupts the therapeutic process.

48) e.
These principles can lead to features like shared decisions and shared activities.

49) e.
The important questions addressed in the framework are (1) 'How does the family function?' (choices **a** to **d** are included in this); and (2) 'Are family factors involved in the patient's problems?' (this is assessed by questions dealing with how the family is reacting, supporting the patient and contributing to the problem).

50) e.
Hypericum perforatum is commonly known as St John's wort; it may cause serotonin toxicity when combined with SSRIs.

51) b.
Risk in the general population is 1/20 000 and there is a 10-fold increase with lithium use.

52) b.
Spina bifida occurs and it is suggested that supplemental folate may reduce the risk.

53) c.
Carbamazepine has a 2.3% risk, lamotrigine 3%, and valproate 7.2%.

54) e.
Atomoxetine can worsen as well as potentially cause angle-closure glaucoma in susceptible individuals.

55) d.
There is a decreased concentration of GABA in the caudate nucleus.

56) c.

The gene is located on chromosome 4; average time to death after diagnosis is 12–16 years; decreased volume of caudate is observed; it causes slowly progressing dementia.

57) e.

General withdrawal and increased muscle tone are also features.

58) a.

The most common infection is *Pneumocystis carinii* pneumonia; dementia is rapidly progressing, with death occurring in 50–75% of cases within 6 months; progression from mild neurocognitive disorder can be prevented by treatment; depression is more common in women than in men.

59) c.

Protease inhibitors induce the metabolism of valproate and alprazolam, and reduce their concentration.

60) e.

Zidovudine and zalcitabine are nucleoside reverse transcriptase inhibitors. Nevirapine and delavirdine are non-nucleoside reverse transcriptase inhibitors. Triple therapy is a combination of two reverse transcriptase inhibitors and a protease inhibitor.

Further reading

British National Formulary. *BNF 57*. London: Pharmaceutical Press. Also available at: www.bnf.org/bnf.

Gelder M, Harrison P, Cowen P. *Shorter Oxford Textbook of Psychiatry*, 5th edn. Oxford: Oxford University Press, 2006.

ICD-10: The ICD-10 Classification of Mental and Behavioural Disorders: Clinical Descriptions and Diagnostic Guidelines. Geneva: World Health Organization, 1990.

Puri B, Hall A. *Revision Notes in Psychiatry*, 2nd edn. London: Arnold/Hodder Education, 2004.

Sadock BJ, Sadock VA. *Kaplan and Sadock's Synopsis of Psychiatry*, 10th edn. Baltimore, MD: Lippincott Williams and Wilkins, 2008.

3. Old age psychiatry: Questions

1) The proportion of people aged above 65 years in the UK according to the figures from the 2001 census was approximately:

   a. 5%
   b. 16%
   c. 1%
   d. 30%
   e. 40%

2) In the UK, among people above the age of 80 the proportion of people having dementia is:

   a. 1 in 5
   b. 1 in 50
   c. 1 in 100
   d. 1 in 1000
   e. 1 in 10 000

3) All of the following are neuropsychological deficits seen in dementia, except:

   a. Amnesia
   b. Alexithymia
   c. Aphasia
   d. Agnosia
   e. Apraxia

4) Which of the following is the most common neuropsychiatric feature seen in dementia?

   a. Hallucinations
   b. Paranoid ideation
   c. Depression
   d. Anxiety
   e. Aggression

5) Which of the following imaging techniques can be used to measure glucose metabolization in different parts of the brain?

   a. CT scan
   b. MR scan
   c. PET scan
   d. SPECT scan
   e. None of the above

6) Which of the following neurotransmitter systems is mainly involved in the mechanism of action of galantamine?

a. Dopamine
b. Noradrenaline
c. Acetylcholine
d. Serotonin
e. Glutamate

7) Which of the following is the main neurotransmitter pathway through which memantine exerts its action?

a. Noradrenaline
b. Acetylcholine
c. Serotonin
d. Histamine
e. Glutamate

8) What are 'Lewy bodies' (the pathological hallmark of dementia with Lewy bodies)?

a. Extracellular neuronal inclusion bodies
b. Intracellular neuronal inclusion bodies
c. Degenerative neuronal products
d. Hyperactivated neuralgia
e. Red-staining senile plaques

9) Which of the following is not an instrument for assessment of cognitive functions?

a. MMSE
b. CDR
c. MBI
d. PANSS
e. ADAS-COG

10) Which of the following statements is not true regarding Pick's disease?

a. It is an autosomal-dominant disease
b. It is primarily a posterior brain pathology
c. It is characterized by loss of pyramidal neurons
d. It is characterized by enlarged lateral ventricles
e. Intracellular inclusion bodies are called Pick bodies

11) Which of the following statements is not true regarding sporadic Creutzfeldt–Jakob disease?

a. It is most commonly seen in people above the age of 80
b. It is the most common form of Creutzfeldt–Jakob disease
c. Dementia is a common presenting feature
d. Histological brain changes are described as spongy in appearance
e. Neurological deficits are common, including ataxia

12) Which of the following is not a gene that has been linked with dementias?

   a. PS-1
   b. PS-2
   c. APOE1
   d. APOE2
   e. NMDA

13) 'Imitation' and 'utilization' behaviours have been described in which of the following syndromes?

   a. Catatonic schizophrenia
   b. Semantic dementia
   c. Dementia with Lewy bodies
   d. Sporadic Creutzfeldt–Jakob disease
   e. Orbitofrontal syndrome

14) In which of the following conditions is the 'fluid void sign' typically seen on imaging?

   a. Alzheimer's disease
   b. Frontotemporal dementia
   c. AIDS-related dementia
   d. Normal-pressure hydrocephalus
   e. Sporadic Creutzfeldt–Jakob disease

15) Which of the following imaging investigations would you avoid in a patient with a cardiac pacemaker while investigating for dementia?

   a. CT scan
   b. MR scan
   c. SPECT scan
   d. PET scan
   e. None of the above

16) In an elderly patient on warfarin, which of the following antidepressants is most likely to interfere with its metabolism?

   a. Fluoxetine
   b. Fluvoxamine
   c. Citalopram
   d. Mianserine
   e. Mirtazapine

17) In an elderly patient, how long a wash-out period would you advise while switching from an SSRI such as citalopram to moclobamide?

   a. No wash-out period
   b. One week
   c. Two weeks
   d. Four weeks
   e. Eight weeks

18) Which of the following scenarios is likely to increase the risk of lithium toxicity in elderly patients?

a. Recurrence of depression
b. Recurrence of mania
c. Concomitant use of antidepressants
d. Concomitant use of diuretics
e. None of the above

19) Which of the following is not a core feature of delirium?

a. Acute onset
b. Fluctuating course
c. Catatonia
d. Perceptual abnormalities
e. Psychomotor disturbance

20) Which of the following terms would best describe the behaviour of a patient with delirium who is aroused, restless, wandersome and pulling repeatedly at the clothing?

a. Confusion
b. Dyspraxia
c. Catatonia
d. Carphologia
e. Aggression

21) Which of the following is not a predisposing factor for delirium?

a. Old age
b. Female sex
c. Visual impairment
d. Immobility
e. Depression

22) Which of the following group of drugs is least likely to cause delirium?

a. SSRIs
b. Tricyclics
c. Tetracyclics
d. Typical antipsychotics
e. Benzodiazepines

23) Which of the following strategies is least likely to help with the management of a patient with delirium on a medical ward?

a. Orientating communication
b. Pain management
c. Movement restriction
d. Avoiding sedation
e. Early discharge

24) Which of the following best indicates the prevalence figures reported in literature for late-life depression

    a. 1–5%
    b. 10–15%
    c. 25%
    d. 35%
    e. 50%

25) What proportion of older people with dementia are expected to have depression?

    a. 5%
    b. 10%
    c. 25%
    d. 50%
    e. Less than 1%

26) Which of the following is not a contributing factor to risk of suicide in older people?

    a. Male gender
    b. Pain
    c. Alcohol abuse
    d. Personality disorder
    e. Residential care

27) The genetic risk of depression in older people is:

    a. The same as in younger adults
    b. Higher than in younger adults
    c. Lower than in younger adults
    d. Significantly higher than in younger adults
    e. No evidence is available

28) Which of the following is the most important risk factor for late-onset depression?

    a. First-degree relatives with depression
    b. Second-degree relatives with depression
    c. Childhood neurotic traits
    d. Cerebrovascular disease
    e. Old age

29) What percentage of people between the ages of 65 and 75 can be considered to be sexually active?

    a. 40%
    b. 20%
    c. 10%
    d. 5%
    e. 1%

30) Approximately what percentage of beds is occupied by people above the age of 65 in a typical general hospital?

a. 15%
b. 25%
c. 40%
d. 50%
e. 75%

31) What is the most common reason for liaison referrals in old age psychiatry?

a. Depression
b. Anxiety disorders
c. Schizophrenia
d. Dementia
e. Alcohol abuse

32) Which of the following statements is true regarding general hospital personnel?

a. They overdiagnose psychiatric illnesses
b. They are good at identifying psychiatric illnesses
c. They are poor at identifying psychiatric illnesses
d. There is no difference from psychiatric services
e. None of the above

33) Which of the following is not true of medically ill patients with delirium?

a. They stay in hospital for a longer time
b. They are less likely to be institutionalized
c. They die sooner
d. They are more likely to have cognitive impairment
e. Complete resolution of delirium is less likely

34) A combination of cognitive impairment and 'alien limb phenomenon' is seen in:

a. Dementia with Lewy bodies
b. Parkinson's disease dementia
c. Frontotemporal dementia
d. Cortical basal degeneration
e. Multisystem atrophy

35) Which of the following syndromes commonly presents with dementia, Parkinsonian symptoms and difficulty in downward gaze?

a. Multiple sclerosis
b. Creutzfeldt–Jakob disease
c. Cortical basal degeneration
d. Progressive supranuclear palsy
e. Normal-pressure hydrocephalus

36) Which illness presents with the classical clinical triad of dementia, myoclonic jerks and periodic EEG?

   a. Dementia with Huntington's disease
   b. Creutzfeldt–Jakob disease
   c. AIDS dementia
   d. Lysosomal disease
   e. Niemann–Pick disease

37) Which of the following statements is not true regarding Wilson's disease?

   a. It is a disorder of copper metabolism
   b. It is autosomal dominant
   c. Kayser–Fleischer rings are a feature
   d. Low serum copper levels are a feature
   e. Elevated urine copper levels are a feature

38) Which of the following symptoms is the least common in late-onset schizophrenia?

   a. Paranoid delusions
   b. Persecutory delusions
   c. Auditory hallucinations
   d. Negative symptoms
   e. Depression

39) Which of the following risk factors is the least important in late-onset schizophrenia?

   a. Family history
   b. Female sex
   c. Paranoid personality traits
   d. Schizoid personality traits
   e. Deafness

40) Which of the following is not an important element of capacity?

   a. Willingness to see the doctor
   b. Understanding the decision to be made
   c. Understanding the alternative choices
   d. Retaining the information
   e. Communicating the decision

41) Which of the following statements is not true regarding the assessment of capacity?

   a. Capacity should be assumed unless proved otherwise
   b. Capacity is specific to a decision
   c. Capacity cannot change in an individual
   d. Capacity can be influenced by communication problems
   e. Undue influence has to be considered

42) Elder abuse most commonly occurs in:

a. The older person's own home
b. On the street
c. In hospital
d. In residential homes
e. In nursing homes

43) The elements of sleep hygiene include all of the following, except:

a. Regular daytime exercise
b. Relaxation techniques
c. Going to bed early in the evening
d. Using the bedroom only for sleep
e. Making the bed as comfortable as possible

44) Which of the following hypnotics could be most useful for early-morning wakefulness in older people?

a. Lorazepam
b. Oxazepam
c. Diazepam
d. Midazolam
e. Chlordiazepoxide

45) Which of the following is not essential for the diagnosis of dementia?

a. Cognitive deficits
b. Functional impairment
c. Clear consciousness
d. Perceptual abnormalities
e. Change from previous level

46) What percentage of all dementia cases is accounted for by Alzheimer's disease?

a. 70–80%
b. 50–60%
c. 30–40%
d. 20–30%
e. 10–20%

47) Which of the following is not a common symptom of frontotemporal dementia?

a. Primitive reflexes
b. Apathy
c. Disinhibition
d. Obsessionality
e. Visual hallucinations

48) Which of the following psychological symptoms is most commonly seen in Alzheimer's disease?

a. Depression
b. Hallucinations
c. Delusions
d. Euphoria
e. Anxiety

49) Which of the following is the most common behavioural symptom of Alzheimer's disease?

a. Apathy
b. Agitation
c. Wandering
d. Physical aggression
e. Verbal aggression

50) Which of the following perceptual abnormalities is most common in Alzheimer's disease?

a. Auditory hallucinations
b. Visual hallucinations
c. Somatic hallucinations
d. Tactile hallucinations
e. Illusions

51) Which of the following is most likely to be effective in treating apathy in Alzheimer's disease?

a. Antidepressants
b. Antipsychotics
c. Anxiolytics
d. Cholinesterase inhibitors
e. ECT

52) Which of the following is not a risk factor for Alzheimer's disease?

a. Age
b. Depression
c. Head injury
d. Male gender
e. Down syndrome

53) What percentage of patients have early-onset (below age 65) Alzheimer's disease?

a. 1%
b. 5%
c. 10%
d. 15%
e. 20%

54) Which of the following is a protective factor for Alzheimer's disease?

a. Down syndrome
b. Apolipoprotein E4 allele
c. Apolipoprotein E2 allele
d. Presenilin-I gene
e. Presenilin-II gene

55) What is the median survival time for Alzheimer's disease?

a. 2–3 years
b. 5–6 years
c. 8–10 years
d. 10–15 years
e. 10 years

56) Abnormal aggregations of which of the following proteins are seen in Lewy bodies?

a. Fibrillar proteins
b. Tau proteins
c. Alpha-synuclein
d. Messenger RNA
e. Transfer RNA

57) Which of the following is not considered a core feature of dementia with Lewy bodies?

a. Fluctuating cognitive deficits
b. Fluctuating functional abilities
c. Persistent visual hallucinations
d. Repeated unexplained falls
e. Parkinsonism

58) Which of the following statements is not true regarding psychotic symptoms in Alzheimer's disease?

a. Use of cholinesterase inhibitors may be beneficial
b. Use of antipsychotics may be beneficial
c. Persistent contradiction of delusional ideas by caregivers may be helpful
d. They may present as misidentifications
e. They may lead to early institutionalization

59) Which of the following symptoms is not commonly seen in the early stage of frontotemporal dementia?

a. Lack of personal and social awareness
b. Lack of judgement
c. Amnesia
d. Reduction in speech output
e. Mental rigidity and inflexibility

60) Which of the following is a common EEG finding in frontotemporal dementia?

a. Abnormal spikes
b. Spike-wave activity
c. Predominant slow-wave activity
d. Mixed spikes and slow-wave activity
e. Normal EEG

61) Which of the following psychotropic medications has the lowest risk of causing delirium?

a. Temazepam
b. Haloperidol
c. Amitriptyline
d. Citalopram
e. Lithium

62) Among older people, the male:female suicide ratio in the UK is:

a. 1:1
b. 2:1
c. 3:1
d. 4:1
e. 5:1

3. Old age psychiatry: Answers

1) b.
The proportion of people aged over 65 was about 16% and is projected to increase to 23% by 2031.

2) a.
About 1 in 5 people aged above 80 in the UK have dementia and about 1 in 20 aged above 65 have dementia.

3) b.
Alexithymia is not a cognitive symptom. It is defined as a person's inability to describe his or her own emotions and mood.

4) c.
Depression is the most common neuropsychiatric feature; some studies have quoted figures of up to 66% of patients having depressive features at some point during their illness.

5) c.
Functional imaging looks at brain function. A PET scan using the ligand fluorodeoxyglucose (FDG) can be used to measure glucose utilization by different parts of the brain. A SPECT scan is generally used to measure the perfusion in different parts of the brain.

6) c.
Galantamine is a reversible inhibitor of acetylcholinesterase and it also has nicotinic receptor agonist properties.

7) e.
Memantine is an NMDA receptor antagonist that affects glutamate transmission.

8) b.
Lewy bodies are intracellular neuronal inclusion bodies that are made up of aggregated filaments of alpha-synuclein.

9) d.
PANSS is the Positive and Negative Syndrome Scale, which is used for schizophrenia.

10) b.
The pathology is frontal and not posterior.

11) a.
Sporadic CJD is usually seen in the fifth and sixth decades.

12) e.
NMDA is a glutamate receptor and not a gene.

13) e.
The orbitofrontal syndrome presents with changes in personality and social interaction characterized by egocentricity, disinhibition and occasionally imitation and utilization.

14) d.
Normal-pressure hydrocephalus.

15) b.
MR scanning should be avoided to prevent the strong magnetic field from interfering with cardiac pacemaker function.

16) b.
The anticoagulant effect is enhanced; the pharmacokinetic interaction is through hepatic cytochrome P450 enzymes.

17) a.
Moclobamide is an RIMA (reversible inhibitor of monoamine oxidase) and has an advantage over conventional MAOIs in that it does not need a wash-out period when switching from an SSRI.

18) d.
Most diuretics are likely to increase the excretion of sodium, which would make elderly people more prone to reduced lithium clearance and at greater risk of toxicity.

19) c.
Catatonia is not considered a core clinical feature of delirium.

20) d.
Carphologia is described in delirium as picking, pulling and grabbing imaginary objects and the patient's own clothes.

21) b.
Male sex is a predisposing factor for delirium.

22) a.
SSRIs act predominantly through the serotonin system, while others have action on the cholinergic system, GABA system, histamine receptors, etc., which are implicated in memory, sedation, etc.

23) c.
Movement restriction can aggravate delirium; physiotherapy is helpful.

24) b.
A range of prevalence figures have been reported for late-life depression with an average figure of 13.5%. Major depression is less common (1–3%).

25) c.
About a quarter of people with dementia develop depressive illness at some point during the course of their illness.

26) e.
Residential care is a protective factor for suicide in older people.

27) c.
The genetic risk is lower in later life. People with late-onset depression have fewer than half as many relatives with a history of depression as people with young-onset depression.

28) d.
Cerebrovascular disease is one of the major risk factors for late-onset depression; the combination has recently been described as vascular depression.

29) b.
20% of people aged 65–75 are sexually active (having intercourse at least once a month).

30) d.
10–25% of people over the age of 65 admitted to medical wards are affected by delirium.

31) d.
The two most common reasons for liaison old age psychiatry referrals are dementia and delirium.

32) c.
A number of studies (see Philpot *et al.* 2005) have shown that general hospital personnel are poor at identifying psychiatric illnesses, especially depression.

Philpot M, Lyons D, Reynolds T. Pages 401–19. *Oxford Textbook of Old Age Psychiatry*. Oxford: Oxford University Press, 2005.

33) b.
Medically ill people with delirium are more likely to be institutionalized on discharge from hospital.

34) d.
Cortical basal degeneration usually presents in late middle or early old age, with akinesia, rigidity, limb apraxia, supranuclear gaze palsy, myoclonus, limb dystonia and cortical sensory loss.

35) d.
Progressive supranuclear palsy presents as an akinetic-rigid syndrome with subcortical dementia; it is also known as Steele–Richardson–Olszewski syndrome.

36) b.
Creutzfeldt–Jakob disease is a very rare form of rapidly progressing dementia; EEG is always abnormal.

37) b.
Wilson's disease is transmitted as an autosomal-recessive trait.

38) d.
Positive symptoms are more common (approximately 46% have at least one first rank symptom). Negative symptoms are the least common.

39) a.
A positive family history is much less common among people with late-onset schizophrenia than among younger people with schizophrenia.

40) a.
A patient might refuse to see a doctor or another professional and yet retain the capacity to make a particular decision.

41) c.
Capacity can vary considerably in an individual over a short space of time, especially in people who are medically ill.

42) a.
The majority of elder abuse occurs in elderly people's own homes.

43) c.
Going to bed early in the evening can lead to late-night sleep disturbance.

44) b.
Oxazepam is considered to be more useful for early-morning wakefulness due to its intermediate half-life. Short-acting benzodiazepines such as lorazepam can be used for sleep-onset problems. Long-acting benzodiazepines such as diazepam and chlordiazepoxide are not recommended for use as hypnotics.

45) d.
Perceptual abnormalities are not essential for the diagnosis of dementia.

46) b.
The most common dementia is Alzheimer's disease, followed by vascular dementia.

47) e.
Visual hallucinations are an unlikely feature of frontotemporal dementia.

48) c.
Delusions are seen in about 30% of cases of Alzheimer's disease.

49) a.
Apathy is the most common behavioural symptom and has been reported in up to 70% of cases.

50) b.
Visual hallucinations are the most common perceptual abnormalities in Alzheimer's disease. About 21% of patients report perceptual abnormalities, of whom 14% have visual hallucinations and about 7% have auditory hallucinations.

51) d.
There is no licensed treatment for apathy in Alzheimer's disease but there is some evidence that cholinesterase inhibitors might be effective.

52) d.
Female gender is one of the possible risk factors for Alzheimer's disease, although it is still not clear whether the higher rates of Alzheimer's disease in females are due to a relatively longer lifespan in women or result from a true risk factor.

53) b.
About 5% of all Alzheimer's disease patients have an early onset and they are likely to have a stronger familial risk.

54) c.
The apolipoprotein E2 allele is a possible protective factor, while the E4 allele is an established risk factor for Alzheimer's disease.

55) b.
A number of studies have shown that the median survival time for Alzheimer's disease (from diagnosis to death) is about 5–6 years.

56) c.

Lewy bodies are primarily made up of aggregates of filamentous alpha-synuclein proteins.

57) d.

Repeated falls, although common in Lewy body dementia, are not considered a core feature.

58) c.

It is usually unhelpful for caregivers of people with Alzheimer's disease to contradict their delusional ideas.

59) c.

Amnesia is rarely seen in the early stages of frontotemporal dementia, which commonly presents with slow onset of deterioration of personality, behaviour and speech.

60) e.

The EEG is normal in the vast majority of cases of frontotemporal dementia.

61) d.

Citalopram and other SSRIs have the lowest risk of causing delirium.

62) d.

Suicide rates increase in elderly people in comparison with the working population. In the UK, about 15% of the population is elderly, but around 25% of suicide occurs in the elderly.

Further reading

Jacoby R, Oppenheimer C, Dening T, Thomas A. *Oxford Textbook of Old Age Psychiatry*. Oxford: Oxford University Press, 2008.

Sheehan B, Karim S, Burns A. *Old Age Psychiatry*. Oxford: Oxford University Press, 2009.

4. Addiction psychiatry and forensic psychiatry: Questions

Addiction psychiatry

1) In the 'stages of change' proposed by Prochaska and DiClemente:

   a. The contemplation stage occurs after the decision stage
   b. The last stage is the maintenance stage
   c. The stage at which the user attempts the change is called the action stage
   d. The action stage occurs before the contemplation stage
   e. The precontemplation stage is when the user accepts that there is a problem and looks at the positive and negative aspects of drug use

2) Which of the following is not a feature of substance dependence as described by Edwards and Gross?

   a. Primacy of drug-seeking behaviour
   b. Widening of drug-taking repertoire
   c. Signs of withdrawal on attempted abstinence
   d. Increased tolerance to the effects of the drug
   e. Rapid reinstatement of previous pattern of drug use after abstinence

3) Which of the following is not equivalent to one unit of alcohol?

   a. Half a pint of 4% beer
   b. One small measure of whisky
   c. One standard glass of 12% wine
   d. One bottle (330 ml) of 4% lager
   e. One small glass of 10% sparkling wine

4) Which of the following statements is false?

   a. The NHS recommends women should not drink more than 2–3 units of alcohol per day on a regular basis
   b. In the UK, roughly 93% of men and 87% of women drink alcohol
   c. In the UK, the legal age for buying alcohol is 18 years
   d. The NHS recommends men should not drink more than 3–4 units of alcohol per day on a regular basis
   e. The lower limit for women is because they have a higher ratio of water to fat than men

5) Regarding the CAGE questionnaire, which of the following statements is true?

   a. It is a screening questionnaire
   b. It asks whether a person feels like cutting back on his or her drinking
   c. There is a question on whether a person feels guilty about his or her drinking
   d. It asks about having a drink early in the morning as an 'eye-opener'
   e. All of the above

6) Which of the following statements is false regarding tests used in alcohol dependence?

   a. The MCV level remains raised for 3–6 months after increased alcohol consumption
   b. A raised γGT level is pathognomic of heavy drinking
   c. Carbohydrate-deficient transferrin level in blood shows around 70% sensitivity
   d. A breath test is useful in assessing recent consumption
   e. The CAGE questionnaire is used for screening

7) Regarding harm reduction, which of the following statements is false?

   a. Motivation is a prerequisite for drug abstinence
   b. Stages of change were described by Prochaska and DiClemente
   c. The maintenance stage is followed by relapse
   d. The contemplation stage is when a user attempts change
   e. The maintenance stage comes after the decision stage

8) All of the following statements are true regarding delirium tremens, except:

   a. There is a reported mortality of 5–10%
   b. It may present with tactile or visual hallucinations
   c. It always occurs in clear consciousness
   d. It can occur even 5 days after the last drink
   e. It is a medical emergency that requires inpatient medical care

9) Regarding maintenance therapy, all of the following statements are true, except:

   a. Disulfiram is usually prescribed once abstinence is achieved
   b. Acamprosate produces an aversive action if taken with alcohol
   c. Naltrexone acts as an anti-craving agent
   d. Naltrexone acts by antagonizing the effects of endogenous endorphins released by alcohol consumption
   e. Disulfiram acts by inhibiting acetaldehyde dehydrogenase

10) Which of the following statements is true of Wernicke–Korsakoff syndrome?

a. The pathology is due to neuronal degeneration following vitamin B6 deficiency
b. It is characterized by a wide-based gait
c. Ophthalmoplegia is due to optic nerve damage
d. With treatment, confusion and ophthalmoplegia are first to resolve
e. People with the syndrome usually have clear consciousness

11) Regarding Korsakoff's psychosis, all of the following statements are true, except:

a. There is significant impairment in the ability to lay down new memories
b. Working memory is unimpaired
c. Procedural memory is grossly impaired
d. It is most commonly caused by thiamine deficiency
e. The presumed mechanism involves a lesion in the mammillothalamic pathway

12) Which of the following is not a medical complication of alcohol misuse?

a. Fatty change in liver
b. Peptic ulceration
c. Gout
d. Tuberculosis
e. All of the above

13) In the UK, what is the percentage of adults who have tried illegal drugs in their lifetime?

a. 10%
b. 20%
c. 33%
d. 80%
e. 65%

14) Which of the following statements is untrue?

a. MDMA is an abbreviation for methyldioxy-N-methamphetamine
b. MDMA causes serotonin release and blocks uptake
c. The 'rush' following MDMA intake lasts for around 3 hours
d. Death can occur after MDMA use, through dehydration and hyperthermia
e. MDMA has hallucinogenic and stimulant properties

15) Which of the following statements is true regarding cocaine intake?

    a. The main route of intake is by injection
    b. Cocaine acts as a cortical depressant
    c. The effect of the drug lasts for a long time because it is metabolized slowly
    d. Cocaine addiction is treated by substitute prescribing
    e. Acute harmful effects include arrhythmia, intense anxiety and hypertension

16) Which of the following statements is false regarding benzodiazepines?

    a. They cause dependency
    b. They are usually taken orally
    c. Temazepam is a short-acting benzodiazepine
    d. They do not cause cross-tolerance with other drugs in the group
    e. They enhance GABA transmission

17) All of the following statements are true regarding LSD, except:

    a. It is a hallucinogen
    b. LSD is an abbreviation for lysergic acid diethylamide
    c. Its use can lead to 'bad trips'
    d. Chronic use leads to flashbacks
    e. Physiological dependence and withdrawal symptoms are very common

18) Which of the following is an immediate effect of cannabis intake?

    a. Depression
    b. Agitation
    c. Low appetite
    d. Bradycardia
    e. Ataxia

19) Which of the following medications has been prescribed for opiate withdrawal?

    a. Lofexidine
    b. Loperamide
    c. Metoclopramide
    d. Ibuprofen
    e. All of the above

20) Which of the following statements is false regarding opiate maintenance therapy?

    a. It should be reviewed daily over the first week of starting therapy
    b. Dose should be increased by 5–10 mg in the first days if needed
    c. Stabilization may take up to 6 weeks
    d. Rapid reduction is achieved within a week
    e. Slow reduction is over a 4- to 6-month period

21) Regarding driving and drug misuse, which of the following statements is false?

a. A conviction for alcohol misuse may incur loss of licence for up to 6 months
b. Alcohol dependence incurs loss of licence for 1 year
c. Dependency on cannabis and LSD may incur loss of licence for 6 months
d. Dependency on heroin or cocaine may incur loss of licence for 3 months
e. Medical screening and a urine test may be required when reinstating a licence

22) Which of the following is an internal trigger to drink?

a. Anxiety
b. View of a pub
c. Smell of alcohol
d. Pressure of work
e. Seeing one's friends drinking

23) Which of the following statements is true regarding motivational interviewing for alcohol addiction?

a. The therapist needs to be highly motivated
b. The patient is encouraged to come up with solutions for his or her drinking problem
c. The therapist gives a choice of solutions to the patient
d. The therapist strongly persuades the patient to stop drinking
e. The patient has only a passive role in the therapy

24) Which of the following statements is true?

a. The setting in which opiate detoxification is carried out affects the outcome
b. There is no evidence base for motivational interviewing in the treatment of drug misuse
c. Advice on safer injecting practices includes using the same injection site
d. A hand signature is always required in controlled drug prescription
e. A shorter-acting opiate is preferred for substitute prescribing

25) Which of the following statements is true regarding cigarette smoking?

a. No difference in prevalence of smoking has been noted between psychosis and neurosis
b. Smoking is less common in lower socioeconomic classes
c. 80% of smokers start before the age of 19
d. Women are more likely than men to smoke cigarettes
e. Most smokers quit after doctor's advice

Forensic psychiatry

26) All of the following can be classed as negligent prescriptions, except:

   a. Failure to treat adverse effects that have or should have been recognized
   b. Unreasonable mixing of drugs
   c. Patient having side-effects from medications prescribed
   d. Prescribing too many drugs at one time
   e. Failing to disclose side-effects of medication

27) Which of the following is an indication for seclusion?

   a. Extremely unstable medical and psychiatric conditions
   b. Overtly suicidal patient
   c. Delirious or demented patient unable to tolerate decreased stimulation
   d. For punishment of the patient, or the convenience of staff
   e. To assist in treatment as part of ongoing behaviour therapy

28) For a person to have capacity, all of the following are necessary, except:

   a. The person should be able to understand the information
   b. The person should be able to believe the information
   c. The person should be able to weigh up the risks and benefits
   d. The person should be able to retain the information for an adequate time
   e. The person should be able to communicate his or her decision

29) Which of the following statements is true regarding a person's fitness to plead?

   a. He or she should be able to comprehend the course of proceedings of the trial, so as to make a proper defence
   b. He or she should know that any jurors to whom he or she may have an objection may be challenged
   c. He or she should be able to comprehend the evidence
   d. He or she should be able to give proper instructions to his or her legal representatives
   e. All of the above

30) What percentage of people guilty of indecent exposure are first-time offenders?

   a. 10%
   b. 20%
   c. 50%
   d. 60%
   e. 80%

31) Which of the following statements is false regarding sexual offences?

   a. Indecent exposure is the most common sexual offence
   b. Female children are victimized more than males
   c. 50% of rapists reoffend sexually
   d. Intrafamilial abuse is usually by father to daughter or step-father to step-daughter
   e. Extrafamilial abuse is less common than intrafamilial

32) What percentage of violent crime in Britain is by people with schizophrenia?

   a. More than 50%
   b. More than 70%
   c. Less than 30%
   d. Less than 50%
   e. Less than 10%

33) Which of the following statements is false?

   a. People with milder forms of learning disability are more likely to offend than those with severe learning disability
   b. Epilepsy is twice as common in offenders as in the general population
   c. Alcohol- and drug-related problems are strongly linked to violence
   d. Depression is commonly associated with violence or aggression
   e. Personality disorder is more strongly related to offending and violence than mental illness

34) Which of the following is not an actuarial risk assessment tool?

   a. HCR-20 (Historical Clinical Risk Management 20)
   b. PCL-R (Psychopathy Checklist–Revised)
   c. VRAG (Violence Risk Appraisal Guide)
   d. ROR (Risk of Reconviction score)
   e. RPS (Reconviction Prediction Score)

35) What percentage of people held in police custody suffer from mental disorder?

   a. 5%
   b. 30%
   c. 50%
   d. 80%
   e. 25%

36) A patient discharged from hospital has been violent and aggressive at home after being non-compliant with his medications. The approved mental health practitioner who went out to see him has not been able to get access to the house. The use of which section of the Mental Health Act would be most appropriate in these conditions?

   a. Section 4
   b. Section 135
   c. Section 2
   d. Section 5(2)
   e. Section 136

37) Regarding crime, which of the following statements is false?

   a. Males between the age of 10 and 20 years account for 50% of crime
   b. Females account for only 20% of offenders
   c. Robbery is one of the most common crimes
   d. Low intelligence is associated with offending
   e. The peak age for committing crime among females is 12–15 years

38) Which of the following statements is true?

   a. Victims of homicide are usually males
   b. Perpetrators of crime are usually females
   c. The majority of homicide offenders are mentally disordered
   d. 5% of victims of homicide are known to offenders
   e. 50% of homicide cases result in a finding of diminished responsibility

39) What percentage of incidents of arson are successfully prosecuted?

   a. 30%
   b. 50%
   c. 15%
   d. 80%
   e. 100%

40) The lifetime risk of violence in people with schizophrenia compared with that in the general population is:

   a. Equal
   b. 50 times higher
   c. 10 times higher
   d. 30 times higher
   e. 5 times higher

41) What percentage of prisoners are transferred to psychiatric hospitals?

a. 45%
b. 5%
c. 25%
d. 75%
e. 15%

42) Which of the following statements is false regarding the MHA 2007?

a. Section 48 allows transfer of mentally disordered sentenced prisoners to hospital
b. Section 47 need reports from two registered medical practitioners
c. Section 41 is a restriction order
d. Section 49 allows the Secretary of State to add a 'restriction direction' to a transfer direction
e. Section 41 is issued by the Crown Court

43) Which of the following statements is false?

a. Diminished responsibility leads to acquittal of the person
b. A person is unfit to stand trial when that person is so unwell that appearance at court would be detrimental to his or her health
c. Fitness to plead is different from fitness to stand trial
d. The Pritchard criteria are used in assessing fitness to plead in England and Wales
e. In a case of a mother killing her baby when the infant is under 12 months old, the court may convict her of infanticide rather than murder

44) In what percentage of domestic violence are women the victim?

a. 10%
b. 25%
c. 50%
d. 70%
e. 85%

45) In which of the following age groups are crime rates highest among males?

a. 22–26 years
b. 14–17 years
c. 30–35 years
d. 38–42 years
e. 50–55 years

46) Which of the following is the most prevalent crime in England and Wales?

a. Sexual offences
b. Robbery
c. Theft
d. Drug offences
e. Violence against another person

47) Which of the following statements is true regarding malpractice? The plaintiff must establish through the evidence that:

a. A doctor–patient relationship existed that created a duty of care
b. There was a deviation from the standard of care
c. The patient was damaged
d. The deviation directly caused the damage
e. All of the above

48) Which of the following statements is true regarding legal automatism?

a. Legal automatism results in increased punishment
b. Night terrors are a type of automatism
c. Sane automatism is caused by intrinsic factors
d. Concussions and dissociative states can lead to insane automatism
e. It is the same as automatism that occurs in complex partial seizures

49) Which of the following statements is false regarding arson?

a. The male:female ratio is 9:1
b. Only a small proportion of arson offences lead to prosecution
c. In patients with psychotic illness, arson is frequently an indirect effect of chronic illness rather than a result of delusions or hallucinations
d. The rate of further arson is 80%
e. The rate of any reoffence is 10–30%

50) Which of the following statements is false regarding exhibitionism?

a. It is commonly seen in younger adults
b. Females are the usual victims
c. Most exhibitionists have low IQ
d. It is different from indecent exposure
e. Flashing and mooning are types of exhibitionism

4. Addiction psychiatry and forensic psychiatry: Answers

1) c.

The stages described by Prochaska and DiClemente are precontemplation, contemplation, decision, action, maintenance and relapse, respectively. Precontemplation is the first of the stages, when a user continues using his or her drug and does not perceive it as a problem. The second stage is contemplation, when a user accepts that there may be a problem. The action stage is when a user attempts to change his or her behaviour. The maintenance stage is when a user continues the abstinence and tries to improve. Relapse is when a user goes back to his or her drug use behaviour.

Prochaska JO, Velicer WF. The transtheoretical model of health behavior change. *Am J Health Promot* 1997; **12**: 38–48.

2) b.

A narrowing of repertoire is seen in drug dependence, when a user moves from a range of drugs to a single drug taken in preference to all others.

Edwards G, Gross MM. Alcohol dependence: provisional description of a clinical syndrome. *Br Med J* 1976; **1**: 1058–61.

3) c.

One standard glass is 175 ml. Hence 12% wine in a standard glass is equivalent to 2.1 units. A pint is 568 ml. One small glass is 125 ml. An easy way to find the number of units is to multiply strength by the volume or measure in ml and divide by 1000.

4) e.

Daily limit has been given more importance. It is recommended that men should have no more than 3–4 units per day and women should have no more than 2–3 units per day. The lower limits for women are due to women's higher ratio of fat to water and hence inability to dilute the alcohol consumed.

5) e.

The CAGE questionnaire is used for screening and consists of questions on Cutting down on drinking, getting Annoyed by people criticizing drinking pattern, feeling Guilty, and using alcohol as an Eye-opener.

6) b.

The γGT level can be raised in other liver diseases, especially chronic diseases. Blood tests are not specific/sensitive enough for routine screening purposes.

7) d.
The stages described by Prochaska and DiClemente are precontemplation, contemplation, decision, action, maintenance and relapse. The contemplation stage is when the user accepts that he or she may have a problem. The user attempts to change at the action stage.

8) c.
Delirium tremens is a medical emergency whereby a person goes into an acute confusional state secondary to alcohol withdrawal. It usually occurs within the first 2 days but can present as many as 7 days after the last drink. Features include clouding of consciousness, disorientation, amnesia for recent events, marked psychomotor agitation and hallucinations.

9) b.
Disulfiram acts as an aversive drug by irreversibly inhibiting acetaldehyde dehydrogenase. Acamprosate and naltrexone act as anti-craving agents. Unlike disulfiram, they do not produce aversive effects if alcohol is consumed with them.

10) d.
Wernicke's encephalopathy is characterized by a classic tetrad of symptoms: acute confusional state, ophthalmoplegia, nystagmus and ataxia. It is due to neuronal degeneration following thiamine (vitamin B1) deficiency. Confusion and ophthalmoplegia are first to resolve.

11) c.
Retrograde amnesia as well as difficulty in laying down new memories is seen. However, procedural memory, emotional memory and working memory are unimpaired. It is presumed that thiamine deficiency causes lesions in the mammillothalamic tract.

12) e.
Most of the systems are affected by alcohol misuse. It also causes erectile dysfunction, foetal alcohol syndrome and osteoporosis.

13) c.
About one-third of the adult population in the UK have tried illegal drugs at least once in their lifetime.

14) a.
MDMA is 3,4,methylenedioxy-N-methamphetamine. It causes serotonin release and blocks uptake. It has hallucinogenic and stimulant properties by potentiating neurotransmission and increasing cortical excitability.

15) e.
Cocaine is a stimulant and has a euphoric action that lasts only for short periods as it is metabolized fast in the body. The main route of intake is by inhalation.

16) d.

Benzodiazepines produce tolerance rapidly with themselves as well as with others in the benzodiazepine group. Their mode of action is by enhancing GABA transmission.

17) e.

LSD is a hallucinogen. Its effect lasts for 6 hours after ingestion. It does not cause physiological dependence or withdrawal symptoms.

18) e.

Cannabis is the most commonly used illegal drug. The immediate effects include euphoria, enhanced sense of well-being, relaxation, increased appetite, mild tachycardia, variable dysarthria and ataxia.

19) e.

Lofexidine is used for hypertension and ibuprofen for headaches and muscle pain.

20) d.

Rapid reduction is achieved in 14–21 days.

21) d.

Dependency on heroin or cocaine may incur loss of licence for 1 year.

22) a.

Anxiety is an internal trigger to drink.

23) b.

In motivational interviewing, the patient plays the active role and is encouraged to find solutions for his or her drinking problem.

24) d.

Research has shown that the setting of opiate detoxification does not affect the outcome. Advice is given to rotate injection sites. Longer-acting opiates like methadone are used in substitute prescribing.

25) c.

Approximately 80% of smokers start smoking before the age of 19 (based on data from the 2006 SAMHSA National Household Survey on Drug Use and Health, available at: www.oas.samhsa.gov/nsduh.htm). Men are more likely to smoke than women. 2% stop smoking within a year after advice from clinicians.

26) c.

The patient needs to be well informed of the side-effects of the medication prescribed, as well as of with the effects. As long as the patient is well informed of the effects and side-effects and monitored for them, a prescription would not be deemed negligent. However, other practices like unreasonable mixing of drugs, or prescribing too many drugs, could be classed as negligent prescription.

27) e.
Seclusion and restraint raise many legal issues and indications need to be documented and discussed. Indications include preventing imminent harm to patient or others, preventing significant disruption to a treatment programme, and decreasing sensory overstimulation. Refer to the forensic psychiatry chapter in Sadock and Sadock (2008).

Sadock BJ, Sadock VA. *Kaplan and Sadock's Synopsis of Psychiatry*, 10th edn. Baltimore, MD: Lippincott Williams and Wilkins, 2008.

28) b.
To have capacity, a person needs to understand, weigh the risks and benefits, retain the information and communicate his or her decision.

29) e.
A person should fulfil Pritchard's criteria to be fit to plead.

30) b.
20% of first-time offenders go on to commit further indecent exposure. 60% of those with previous sexual offences and 70% with previous sexual and non-sexual offences commit further indecent exposure.

Semple D, Smyth R. *Oxford Handbook of Psychiatry*, 2nd edn. Oxford: Oxford University Press, 2009.

31) c.
The rate of reoffending among sex offenders is low. Only 15% of rapists reoffend sexually and 20% commit violent non-sexual offences.

Semple D, Smyth R. *Oxford Handbook of Psychiatry*, 2nd edn. Oxford: Oxford University Press, 2009.

32) e.
People with schizophrenia account for less than 10% of all violent crimes in Britain.

Semple D, Smyth R. Forensic psychiatry. In: *Oxford Handbook of Psychiatry*, 2nd edn. Oxford: Oxford University Press, 2009.

33) d.
Depression is very rarely associated with violence or offending. Affective disorders are less commonly associated with offending and violence than schizophrenia. Milder forms of learning disability are more common than severe learning disability in this group of patients. The offences are

broadly similar to offences by people without learning disabilities and are more due to family and social disadvantage. Epilepsy is more prevalent, while violence from epileptic activity is very rare.

Semple D, Smyth R. *Oxford Handbook of Psychiatry*, 2nd edn. Oxford: Oxford University Press, 2009.

34) a.
Risk assessment tools can be either structured clinical or actuarial. The HCR-20 is a structured clinical tool, while all the others are actuarial tools. Structured clinical tools combine the historical factors of the actuarial approach with dynamic factors in a structured way.

Semple D, Smyth R. *Oxford Handbook of Psychiatry*, 2nd edn. Oxford: Oxford University Press, 2009.

35) a.
2–5% of people held in police custody suffer from mental disorder. Only 1–2% suffer from severe mental illness.

Semple D, Smyth R. *Oxford Handbook of Psychiatry*, 2nd edn. Oxford: Oxford University Press, 2009.

36) b.
The approved mental health practitioner should apply for a section 135 for the police to break into the patient's house and bring him to the hospital or nearest place of safety. Section 4 is used in emergencies when a second doctor is not available. Section 2 is used for assessment for 28 days. Section 5(2) is doctors' holding power for 72 hours. Section 136 gives the police power to remove a person appearing to have a mental disorder from a public place to a place of safety for the person's or pubic safety.

37) c.
Robbery is one of the rarest forms of crime. The most common ones are theft, burglary, criminal damage and car crime.

Semple D, Smyth R. *Oxford Handbook of Psychiatry*, 2nd edn. Oxford: Oxford University Press, 2009.

38) a.
About 70% of homicide victims are males. Males (80–90%) are the main perpetrators of crime. Only a minority of homicide offenders have a mental disorder. 60–80% of victims are known to offenders. 5–10% of cases result in a finding of diminished responsibility.

39) c.

Less than 20% of cases of arson lead to prosecution. Rates of further arson are around 2–20%.

Semple D, Smyth R. *Oxford Handbook of Psychiatry*, 2nd edn. Oxford: Oxford University Press, 2009.

40) e.

The lifetime risk of violence in people with schizophrenia is five times greater than in the general population. People with schizophrenia account for less than 10% of all violent crime in Britain.

Semple D, Smyth R. *Oxford Handbook of Psychiatry*, 2nd edn. Oxford: Oxford University Press, 2009.

41) b.

About 2–5% of prisoners are transferred to psychiatric hospital. About 23–55% of prisoners have psychiatric needs.

42) a.

Section 47 allows transfer of a mentally disordered sentenced prisoner to hospital and needs reports from two medical practitioners addressing the category of mental disorder and whether it is of a nature and degree to warrant hospital admission. Section 48 is similar to section 47 but deals with unsentenced prisoners. Section 41 is issued by the Crown Court and is a restriction order.

43) a.

Diminished responsibility may lead to conviction for the lesser offence of manslaughter but does not result in acquittal.

44) d.

70% of incidents of domestic violence have women as the victim.

Semple D, Smyth R. *Oxford Handbook of Psychiatry*, 2nd edn. Oxford: Oxford University Press, 2009.

45) b.

Males aged 10–20 years account for 50% of crimes. The peak age of offending is between 14 and 17 years.

46) c.

Theft is the most common crime (about 41% of all crime) in England and Wales. Sexual offences and robbery (theft with violence or intimidation) are less frequent.

47) e.

The plaintiff (i.e. the patient) or his or her family or estate must establish that there existed a doctor–patient relationship, that there was a deviation of standard care, that the patient was damaged and that the deviation directly caused the damage.

Sadock BJ, Sadock VA. *Kaplan and Sadock's Synopsis of Psychiatry*, 10th edn. Baltimore, MD: Lippincott Williams and Wilkins, 2008.

48) b.

Legal automatisms result in decreased punishment and even acquittal. Sane automatism is due to extrinsic factors, while insane is due to intrinsic factors. It is different from the concept of automatism in complex partial seizures.

49) d.

The rate of further acts of arson is 2–20%. Males most commonly commit arson offences. Less than 20% of offences lead to prosecution.

50) c.

Most have a normal IQ. Exhibitionism is more commonly seen in young adults than in elderly people. Young girls are the usual victims.

Further reading

British National Formulary. *BNF 57*. London: Pharmaceutical Press. Also available at: www.bnf.org/bnf.

Gelder M, Harrison P, Cowen P. *Shorter Oxford Textbook of Psychiatry*, 5th edn. Oxford: Oxford University Press, 2006.

ICD-10: The ICD-10 Classification of Mental and Behavioural Disorders: Clinical Descriptions and Diagnostic Guidelines. Geneva: World Health Organization, 1990.

Puri B, Hall A. *Revision Notes in Psychiatry*, 2nd edn. London: Arnold/ Hodder Education, 2004.

Sadock BJ, Sadock VA. *Kaplan and Sadock's Synopsis of Psychiatry*, 10th edn. Baltimore, MD: Lippincott Williams and Wilkins, 2008.

Semple D, Smyth R. *Oxford Handbook of Psychiatry*, 2nd edn. Oxford: Oxford University Press, 2009.

5. Child and adolescent psychiatry and learning disability: Questions

Child and adolescent psychiatry

1) Which of the following statements is false regarding attention deficit hyperactivity disorder (ADHD)?

   a. It is more prevalent in males
   b. Behaviour should occur in at least two settings
   c. Behaviour should persist for at least 3 months
   d. It has an incidence of around 1% in the UK
   e. About 20% of children with ADHD develop dissocial personality traits

2) Which of the following statements is false regarding Ritalin (methylphenidate)?

   a. Its mechanism of action is by increasing release of dopamine and noradrenaline
   b. It increases appetite and weight
   c. Tolerance to it may develop over time
   d. It enhances growth
   e. Growth suppression may be prevented with drug holidays

3) Conduct disorder includes all of the following, except:

   a. Cruelty to animals
   b. Aggression to humans
   c. Destruction of property
   d. Theft
   e. Obeying rules

4) Which of the following statements is true regarding oppositional defiant disorder?

   a. It is more common in girls
   b. Onset is after 1 year of age
   c. Behaviour should be seen in two or more situations
   d. It is characterized by serious violation of societal laws
   e. 25% of children with the disorder show no symptoms in later life

5) Which of the following is not a pervasive developmental disorder?

   a. Rett syndrome
   b. ODD
   c. PDD-NOS
   d. Asperger syndrome
   e. Autism

6) Which of the following statements is false regarding Asperger syndrome?

   a. It is more common in males
   b. Depression is a very common feature
   c. Deficits in social, language and behavioural skills present
   d. Family history of autism presents
   e. Schizophrenia is more common in children with Asperger syndrome than in the general population

7) Which of the following statements is true regarding children with attention deficit hyperactivity disorder (ADHD)?

   a. Learning disability is very rare with ADHD
   b. Children with ADHD are good at task completion
   c. Connor's Assessment Scale is used in ADHD
   d. Cognitive behavioural therapy is not effective
   e. ADHD is seen only in children

8) Regarding conduct disorder, all of the following statements are true, except:

   a. It is more common in boys than girls
   b. Less than 50% of children with the disorder have severe and persistent antisocial problems
   c. Children with poor parenting and low socioeconomic status have a poor prognosis
   d. Children with the disorder usually have a high IQ
   e. Cognitive behavioural therapy and family therapy are helpful in management

9) What percentage of autistic children suffer from learning disability?

   a. 20%
   b. 30%
   c. 50%
   d. 70%
   e. 5%

10) Which of the following statements is false regarding autism?

   a. It is characterized by abnormal social relatedness
   b. Onset of symptoms usually occurs after age 3
   c. Restricted, repetitive and stereotyped behaviour is typical
   d. It is more prevalent in males
   e. One-third of children with autism have increased serum serotonin levels

11) What percentage of children in the UK have a reading disorder?

    a. 4%
    b. 2%
    c. 10%
    d. 15%
    e. 20%

12) Which of the following statements is true regarding enuresis?

    a. It is more common in females
    b. It is usually diagnosed in the first year of birth
    c. No family history has been noted
    d. Behavioural modification is the mainstay of treatment
    e. It results in high self-esteem

13) Concerning Gilles de la Tourette syndrome, which of the following statements is false?

    a. It is characterized by motor and vocal tics
    b. Its prevalence is around 5 per 10 000
    c. It is usually associated with obsessive compulsive disorder
    d. Psycho-education and cognitive behavioural therapy have been found to be helpful
    e. It does not cause distress or affect functioning

14) Which of the following statements is false regarding major depression in children?

    a. Risk of suicide is high
    b. There is a prevalence of up to 3% in prepubescent children
    c. 20% of these children later manifest bipolar disorder as adults
    d. It is prevalent more in males in the adolescent age group
    e. Psychotherapy is the treatment of choice

15) Which of the following statements is true of schizophrenia in children?

    a. There is a better prognosis than in adults
    b. It has a more insidious onset
    c. About 70% later receive a diagnosis of bipolar disorder or schizoaffective disorder
    d. It responds well to treatment
    e. Delusion is the most common symptom

16) A 10-year-old boy has been diagnosed as suffering from attention deficit hyperactivity disorder, with no comorbidity. The family have tried psychotherapy and want to know about any pharmacological interventions. Which would be the drug of choice in this condition?

a. Imipramine
b. Fluoxetine
c. Methylphenidate
d. Desipramine
e. Atomoxetine

17) Regarding hyperkinetic disorder, which of the following statements is true?

a. It may be diagnosed by a GP
b. It can be diagnosed through rating scales alone
c. Attention deficit hyperactivity disorder should be considered in all age groups
d. It can be diagnosed even if the history shows that it is prevalent only in one setting
e. Dietary fatty acid supplements are recommended for treatment

18) National Institute for Health and Clinical Excellence (NICE) recommendations for depression in children include all of the following, except:

a. Drugs are not recommended as the first-line treatment in mild depression
b. Psychotherapy is the first-line treatment for moderate to severe depression
c. Medication should be offered in combination with psychotherapy
d. The preferred antidepressant is fluoxetine, after a course of psychotherapy has been tried
e. A child when initially diagnosed with mild depression should be referred to tier 4 CAMHS

19) What percentage of children and young people suffer from obsessive compulsive disorder?

a. 1%
b. 5%
c. 8%
d. 10%
e. 15%

20) A 7-year-old boy has been diagnosed with severe obsessive compulsive disorder, with no comorbidity. Psychotherapy has been tried with not much benefit. The multidisciplinary team has discussed treatment with his family and has agreed on trying pharmacological intervention. Which is the medication of choice according to National Institute for Health and Clinical Excellence (NICE) guidelines?

a. Fluoxetine
b. Sertraline
c. Fluvoxamine
d. Tricyclics
e. Methylphenidate

21) Which is the drug of choice in attention deficit hyperactivity disorder with conduct disorder?

a. Atomoxetine
b. Risperidone
c. Methylphenidate
d. Fluoxetine
e. Clonidine

22) Which of the following statements is true of atomoxetine?

a. It is the drug of choice in attention deficit hyperactivity disorder with no comorbid symptoms according to National Institute for Health and Clinical Excellence (NICE) guidelines
b. It does not have any gastric side-effects
c. It is a stimulant medication
d. It works as a noradrenaline reuptake inhibitor
e. It is not approved for use in adults

23) Which of the following statements is false regarding autism?

a. Age of onset is before 38 months
b. There is a preponderance in males
c. Communication difficulties present
d. It is characterized by lack of friends
e. Autistic children usually have a high IQ

24) In Rett syndrome, all of the following statements are true, except:

a. Prenatal and perinatal development is normal
b. Head circumference at birth is normal
c. It is seen only in girls
d. There is acceleration of head growth between 5 and 48 months
e. Gait and trunk movements are poorly coordinated

25) Which of the following is not a feature of attention deficit hyperactivity disorder?

a. Being physically cruel to animals
b. Failure to sustain attention during a task
c. Leaving one's seat in a classroom when expected to sit down
d. Blurting out the answer before questions are completed
e. Talking excessively without appropriate response to social constraints

Learning disability

26) What percentage of learning disability is due to prenatal factors?

a. 70%
b. 20%
c. 35%
d. 90%
e. 5%

27) Which of the following statements is false regarding Down syndrome?

a. It is the most common genetic cause of learning disability
b. It is due to trisomy of chromosome 21
c. Children with Down syndrome have characteristic facies and habitus
d. Learning disability is evident before the age of 1 year
e. IQ in adults is usually less than 50

28) Which of the following statements is true regarding Patau syndrome?

a. It is due to trisomy of chromosome 17
b. Children with the syndrome may have rocker-bottom feet
c. Children with the syndrome have normal genitalia
d. IQ is usually normal
e. It is caused only by non-disjunction of chromosomes during meiosis

29) Which of the following statements is false regarding Down syndrome?

a. Incidence per 1000 live births increases for women over 35
b. Raised IgM and IgG levels are features
c. The usual genetic cause is a Robertsonian translocation
d. Most children with Down syndrome are born to mothers under the age of 35
e. About half of people with Down syndrome have congenital heart defects

30) All of the following diseases in the mother during pregnancy can lead to learning disability, except:

a. Diabetes
b. Hypothyroidism
c. Syphilis
d. German measles
e. Measles

31) People with Down syndrome have an increased risk of:

a. Vascular dementia
b. Hyperthyroidism
c. Depression
d. Hypermetropia
e. Macrocephaly

32) Which of the following is not a feature of Down syndrome?

a. High-arched palate
b. Short stature
c. Protruding tongue
d. Kayser–Fleischer ring
e. Simian crease

33) With which of the following syndromes is learning disability rarely associated?

a. Down syndrome
b. Turner syndrome
c. Trisomy X
d. Klinefelter syndrome
e. XYY male

34) Prader–Willi syndrome consists of all of the following, except:

a. Acromicria
b. Hypogenitalism
c. Tall stature
d. Mild to moderate learning disability
e. Obesity

35) Which of the following is a feature of Angelman syndrome?

a. Paroxysms of crying
b. Macrocephaly
c. Micrognathia
d. Epilepsy
e. Normal IQ

36) Which of the following statements is true regarding phenylketonuria?

   a. It is an unpreventable cause of learning disability
   b. It can be detected by the Widal test
   c. It can be treated by external supply of phenylalanine
   d. It is caused by a defect on the short arm of chromosome 12
   e. Behaviour symptoms include temper tantrums and hyperactivity

37) Which of the following statements is true regarding fragile X syndrome?

   a. It shows a triplet sequence of CCG
   b. It is transmitted as X-linked recessive
   c. It does not occur in females
   d. It is the most common inherited cause of learning disability
   e. It has very high penetrance

38) Which of the following is associated with tall stature?

   a. Down syndrome
   b. XYY
   c. Foetal alcohol syndrome
   d. Prader–Willi syndrome
   e. Hunter syndrome

39) Which of the following is associated with microcephaly?

   a. Down syndrome
   b. Cri-du-chat
   c. Hurler syndrome
   d. Hydrocephalus
   e. Fragile X

40) The clinical picture of congenital hypothyroidism includes all of the following, except:

   a. Hyperactivity
   b. Feeding difficulty
   c. Constipation
   d. Macroglossia
   e. Umbilical hernia

41) Which one of the following disorders would benefit from dietary restriction?

   a. Down syndrome
   b. Sturge–Weber syndrome
   c. Phenylketonuria
   d. Hunter syndrome
   e. Fragile X syndrome

42) What is the prevalence of epilepsy in hospitalized patients with learning disability?

a. 10%
b. 25%
c. 80%
d. 40%
e. 60%

43) Which of the following statements is false regarding psychiatric diseases in individuals with learning disability?

a. Age of onset of schizophrenia tends to be earlier than in the general population
b. Genetic factors are important in the aetiology of schizophrenia
c. Bipolar disorder is less prevalent than in the general population
d. Suicidal thoughts are less frequent in individuals with severe learning disability than in those with mild/moderate learning disability
e. Anxiety disorders are difficult to differentiate from depression

44) Which of the following statements is true regarding behaviour disorders in individuals with learning disability?

a. Self-injurious behaviour is less common in severe learning disability
b. 'Self-hugging' stereotypic behaviour is seen in Lesch–Nyhan syndrome
c. In Smith–Magenis syndrome clients show a hand-flapping stereotype
d. Behavioural disorder prevalence is around 7% of the population with learning disability
e. Behavioural disorders are less prevalent in inpatients than in the community

45) Which of the following statements is false regarding the DSM-IV classification of mental retardation?

a. Adults with mild mental retardation can live independently with appropriate support and raise their own families
b. Moderate mental retardation is the most frequent type of mental retardation
c. Children with profound mental retardation may be taught some self-care skills
d. Most children with moderate mental retardation acquire language and can communicate adequately during early childhood
e. The cause of severe mental retardation is more likely to be identified than the causes of other milder forms

46) Which of the following statements is false regarding children with Smith–Magenis syndrome?

a. They usually have mild mental retardation
b. They present with self-injury behaviour like head-banging and hand-biting
c. They have decreased REM sleep
d. Their voice is usually hoarse and deep
e. The syndrome is caused by complete or partial deletion of 17p11

47) Which of the following statements is true regarding tuberous sclerosis?

   a. It is an autosomal-recessive condition
   b. More than 80% of patients have learning disability
   c. The cancerous growths seen are known as hamartomas
   d. It is caused by deletion on chromosome 5
   e. There may be associated developmental delay

48) Which of the following statements is true regarding Angelman syndrome?

   a. It usually presents with macrocephaly
   b. It is caused by inactivation of paternally inherited chromosome 15
   c. It is named after the first patient diagnosed with the syndrome
   d. Characteristic patterns are seen on EEG
   e. Speech development is normal

49) Which of the following statements is false?

   a. Folic-acid supplementation during early pregnancy reduces the prevalence of learning disability
   b. Maternal illnesses like diabetes can lead to learning disability
   c. Urinary tract infection (UTI) in the mother during pregnancy leads to learning disability in the child
   d. Neonatal screening for hypothyroidism prevents learning disability
   e. Central nervous system infections in the first year of life can lead to learning disability

50) Which of the following statements is false regarding Rett syndrome?

   a. Symptoms can be seen from the first month of life
   b. It exclusively affects girls
   c. It is often associated with autism
   d. Self-injury presents in 40–50% of patients
   e. Epilepsy is a common feature

5. Child and adolescent psychiatry and learning disability: Answers

1) c.
To diagnose ADHD, the inattention and/or hyperactivity should be present in at least two settings and should persist for at least 6 months.

2) b.
Methylphenidate is used in attention deficit hyperactivity disorder and narcolepsy. It increases concentration and decreases impulsivity. Growth suppression is a concerning side-effect, which can be reduced by having 'drug holidays'.

3) e.
Conduct disorder includes cruelty to animals, aggression to humans, destruction of property, disregard of rules, deceitfulness and theft.

4) e.
Oppositional defiant disorder has onset between 3 and 8 years. It is more common in boys but prevalence is equal in adolescents. Children show negative and hostile behaviour but do not break rules or violate the rights of others.

5) b.
Pervasive developmental disorders (PDDs) are disorders with deficits in social, communication and behavioural skills. They are usually associated with autism.

6) c.
Asperger syndrome is considered in the same spectrum as autism. One of the main differences is that language skills are not affected in Asperger syndrome.

7) c.
60% of people with ADHD have learning disability. Because of poor attention spans, they are usually bad at task completion. Cognitive behavioural therapy is found to be effective. ADHD is also seen in teenagers and adults.

8) d.
Children with conduct disorder have low IQ. It is more common in boys. Low cerebrospinal fluid serotonin levels, low IQ and brain injury are biological factors associated with risk of conduct disorder.

9) d.
70% of autistic children suffer from mild to moderate learning disability.

10) b.
In autism, symptoms usually appear before the age of 3. Autism is characterized by abnormal social relatedness, qualitative abnormality in communication and restricted, repetitive and stereotyped behaviour.

11) a.
4% of school-age children have difficulty in reading. A male predominance has been noted.

Semple D, Smyth R. *Oxford Handbook of Psychiatry*, 2nd edn. Oxford: Oxford University Press, 2009.

12) d.
Enuresis is micturition in a child of 5 years or more, usually at night. This could be voluntary or involuntary. Usually there is a family history. It is more common in males and results in low self-esteem. Imipramine may be used if behavioural management does not work.

13) e.
Gilles de la Tourette syndrome is characterized by motor and vocal tics. It causes distress and impaired functioning.

14) d.
Major depression has an equal gender ratio in prepubescent children. However, in adolescent groups prevalence is 8% for males and 14% for females.

15) b.
Schizophrenia in children has a poor prognosis, an insidious onset and responds poorly to treatment. Delusions and catatonia are rare. Only 30% of children receive a diagnosis of schizoaffective disorder or bipolar disorder in later life.

16) c.
The drug of choice in ADHD with no comorbidity, according to National Institute for Health and Clinical Excellence (NICE) guidelines, is methylphenidate. It has to be started at a low dose and titrated weekly.

17) c.
According to National Institute for Health and Clinical Excellence (NICE) guidelines, hyperkinetic disorder should be considered in all age groups. It should be diagnosed by specialists or professionals with appropriate training and expertise. It should not be diagnosed from rating scales or observational data alone. The symptoms should also be present in at least two settings for the diagnosis to be made. Dietary fatty acid supplementation is not recommended.

18) e.
Refer to National Institute for Health and Clinical Excellence (NICE) guidelines on depression in children and young people. Mild depression should be referred to tier 1 in the first instance. No medication is recommended for mild depression.

National Institute for Health and Clinical Excellence. *Depression: Management of Depression in Primary and Secondary Care – NICE Guidance*. London: NICE, 2004. Available at: www.nice.org.uk/CG023.

19) a.
About 1% of children and young people suffer from obsessive compulsive disorder, according to National Institute for Health and Clinical Excellence (NICE) guidelines.

National Institute for Health and Clinical Excellence. *Obsessive-Compulsive Disorder: Core Interventions in the Treatment of Obsessive-Compulsive Disorder and Body Dysmorphic Disorder*. London: NICE, 2005. Available at: www.nice.org.uk/Guidance/CG31.

20) b.
Sertraline is the drug of choice according to National Institute for Health and Clinical Excellence (NICE) guidelines. Sertraline and fluvoxamine are preferred in obsessive compulsive disorder with no comorbid symptoms. However, fluvoxamine is authorized only in children above 8 years old.

National Institute for Health and Clinical Excellence. *Depression: Management of Depression in Primary and Secondary Care – NICE Guidance*. London: NICE, 2004. Available at: www.nice.org.uk/CG023.

21) c.
The National Institute for Health and Clinical Excellence (NICE) recommends methylphenidate in children with ADHD with conduct disorder.

22) d.
Atomoxetine is a noradrenaline reuptake inhibitor used in ADHD. It can be used in children and adults. The most common side-effects include nausea and vomiting.

23) e.
About 70% of autistic children have low IQ. The male:female ratio is 3–4:1.

24) d.
Rett syndrome is seen only in girls. There is normal growth until 5 months, then from 6 months there is deceleration of head growth.

25) a.
Cruelty and aggression to animals and people are part of conduct disorder.

26) a.
50–70% of cases are due to prenatal factors, 10–20% to perinatal and another 5–10% to postnatal factors.

27) d.
Although Down syndrome is diagnosed at birth, learning disability becomes evident only by the end of the first year.

28) b.
Patau syndrome is due to trisomy of chromosome 13. Children with Patau syndrome have abnormal genitalia and low IQ. It can be caused by other malfunctions like translocation.

29) c.
The most common cause of Down syndrome is trisomy 21 (more than 95% of cases). Only less than 5% is due to a Robertsonian translocation. The incidence per 1000 live births increases greatly from 5 in women under 35 to 25 in women under 40 years, but because of the higher number of pregnancies in younger women, most children with Down syndrome are born to mothers under the age of 35 years.

30) e.
Learning disability in a baby can be caused by the mother suffering from one of the following illnesses: non-infectious causes are diabetes, hypothyroidism, hypertension and malnutrition; infectious causes include syphilis, HIV and TORCH (toxoplasmosis, rubella, cytomegalovirus, herpes simplex) (rubella is German measles).

31) c.
Down syndrome patients have an increased risk of Alzheimer's dementia, hypothyroidism (20%), depression (10%), myopia (30%) and brachycephaly.

32) d.
Kayser–Fleischer rings are dark rings that are seen around the iris in copper poisoning. The eye manifestation seen in Down syndrome is Brushfield spots, which are grey or very light yellow spots on the iris.

33) b.
Turner syndrome does not typically cause learning disability. Males with XYY may have slightly lower than average IQ.

34) c.

Features of Prader–Willi syndrome include short stature, hypogenitalism (cryptorchidism, micropenis, amenorrhoea), overeating, obesity, mild to moderate learning disability and sleep disorders.

Semple D, Smyth R. *Oxford Handbook of Psychiatry*, 2nd edn. Oxford: Oxford University Press, 2009.

35) d.

Angelman (happy puppet) syndrome features ataxia, epilepsy (86%), paroxysms of laughter, microcephaly, prominent jaw and severe or profound learning disability.

36) e.

Phenylketonuria is a preventable cause of learning disability. It is due to deficiency of phenylalanine hydroxylase. The gene for phenylalanine hydroxylase is located on the long arm of chromosome 12. It is detected postnatally by the Guthrie test. Management consists of restriction of phenylalanine.

37) d.

Fragile X syndrome is the most common inherited cause of learning disability. It has low penetrance. It can occur in both sexes. It is an X-linked dominant condition and shows a repeat of the CGG nucleotide.

38) b.

All are associated with short stature except XYY. Other syndromes that feature tall stature are XXY and fragile X.

39) b.

Cri-du-chat syndrome is caused by a deletion on chromosome 5. It is usually sporadic. It causes a cat-like cry, microcephaly and a rounded face. It is usually associated with severe or profound learning disability.

40) a.

Congenital hypothyroidism is a treatable cause of mental and growth retardation. The typical clinical picture in an untreated case is one of lethargy, feeding difficulty, constipation, macroglossia and umbilical hernia.

41) c.

Dietary restriction of phenylalanine may improve prognosis in phenylketonuria.

42) d.

The prevalence of epilepsy in the hospitalized learning-disabled population is 40%.

Semple D, Smyth R. *Oxford Handbook of Psychiatry*, 2nd edn. Oxford: Oxford University Press, 2009.

43) c.

The age of onset of schizophrenia tends to be earlier in learning disability than in the general population (mean 23 years). Mood disorders are more prevalent in learning disability, but suicidal thoughts may be less prevalent in the severely disabled. It is usually difficult to differentiate anxiety disorders from depression.

44) d.

Self-injurious behaviour is more common with severe learning disability. Behavioural disorders are more prevalent (two to three times) in inpatients than in the community. Learning-disabled patients with genetic aetiology may have characteristic behaviour stereotypes. In Smith–Magenis syndrome, they show 'self-hugging' behaviour. Hand-flapping is seen in fragile X syndrome.

45) b.

Mild mental retardation is the most frequent type of mental retardation (85%). Many adults can live independently with appropriate support and raise their own families. Moderate mental retardation is the second most prevalent (10%). People with moderate mental retardation acquire knowledge and can communicate adequately during early childhood. Severe mental retardation occurs in 4% and the cause of the mental retardation can be identified more readily than in milder cases. Such people may adapt well to supervised living situations such as group homes and also manage to perform work-related tasks under supervision. Profoundly mentally retarded persons represent around 1–2%. They may be taught some self-care skills and learn to communicate their needs given the appropriate training.

Sadock BJ, Sadock VA. *Kaplan and Sadock's Synopsis of Psychiatry*, 10th edn. Baltimore, MD: Lippincott Williams and Wilkins, 2008.

46) a.

Smith–Magenis syndrome presents with severe mental retardation. The syndrome is caused by complete or partial deletion of 17p11. People with Smith–Magenis syndrome show hyperactivity and self-injury behaviour and their voice is deep and hoarse.

47) e.

Tuberous sclerosis is an autosomal-dominant condition with 100% penetrance. It is a multisystemic genetic disease with two genetic loci, on chromosomes 9 and 16. Around 50% suffer from learning disability (Ridler *et al.* 2007). The benign growths are called hamartomas, while the cancerous ones are known as hamartoblastomas.

Ridler K, Suckling J, Higgins NJ, de Vries PJ, Stephenson CM, Bolton PF, Bullmore ET. Neuroanatomical correlates of memory deficits in tuberous sclerosis complex. *Cereb Cortex* 2007; **17**: 261–71.

48) d.

Angelman syndrome is named after Dr Harry Angelman, the British doctor who first described the illness. It is caused by deletion of the maternally inherited chromosome 15. Usual presentation includes developmental delay, speech impairment, ataxia and repetitive behaviour. Other common features include microcephaly, seizures and abnormal EEG.

49) c.

Folic-acid supplementation reduces learning disability. The mother having a UTI during pregnancy has not been seen to cause learning disability in the baby.

50) a.

Rett syndrome is exclusively seen in girls; development is normal until 18–24 months. Associated features include autism, epilepsy and abnormal involuntary movement. Behavioural symptoms include low mood, anxiety and self-injury.

Further reading

British National Formulary. *BNF 57*. London: Pharmaceutical Press. Also available at: www.bnf.org/bnf.

Gelder M, Harrison P, Cowen P. *Shorter Oxford Textbook of Psychiatry*, 5th edn. Oxford: Oxford University Press, 2006.

ICD-10: The ICD-10 Classification of Mental and Behavioural Disorders: Clinical Descriptions and Diagnostic Guidelines. Geneva: World Health Organization, 1990.

Puri B, Hall A. *Revision Notes in Psychiatry*, 2nd edn. London: Arnold/Hodder Education, 2004.

Sadock BJ, Sadock VA. *Kaplan and Sadock's Synopsis of Psychiatry*, 10th edn. Baltimore, MD: Lippincott Williams and Wilkins, 2008.

Semple D, Smyth R. *Oxford Handbook of Psychiatry*, 2nd edn. Oxford: Oxford University Press, 2009.

6. Research methods, evidence-based practice, statistics and critical appraisal 1: Questions

1) Which of the following statements is not true regarding relative risk?

    a. It is also called risk ratio
    b. It compares the risk of disease and death in two groups
    c. The 'exposed' group is the group of prime interest
    d. The 'unexposed' group is the comparison group
    e. A relative risk greater than 1.0 indicates a decreased risk for the 'exposed' group

2) If...

    A = number of people with disease and exposure
    B = number of people without disease but with exposure
    C = number of people with disease but without exposure
    D = number of people without disease and without exposure,

which of the following equations will calculate the odds ratio?

    a. AB divided by CD
    b. AC divided by BD
    c. AA divided by BD
    d. AD divided by BC
    e. ABD divided by ACB

3) Which of the following statements is not true regarding a placebo drug used in a clinical trial?

    a. It has no effect
    b. It is pharmacologically inert
    c. It is identical in appearance to the active drug
    d. The person administering the drug is blinded
    e. It should be given with as much confidence as the active drug

4) Which of the following factors is least likely to influence the placebo effect of a particular drug?

    a. Size of the tablet
    b. Colour of the tablet
    c. Status of the person administering the drug
    d. Age of the patient
    e. Expectation of the patient

5) Which of the following statements is true regarding measures of central location?

   a. They are a range of values that best represent a characteristic of a group of individuals
   b. They are a single value that best represent a characteristic of a group of individuals
   c. They are a measure that quantifies how much individuals in a group vary from each other
   d. They are a measure that quantifies how much individuals in a group vary from other groups
   e. None of the above

6) Which of the following is not a measure of central tendency?

   a. Arithmetic mean
   b. Median
   c. Mode
   d. Range
   e. Mid-range

7) Which of the following describes the normal distribution?

   a. Symmetric
   b. Asymmetric
   c. Skewed
   d. Positively skewed
   e. Negatively skewed

8) All of the following statements are true regarding the 'arithmetic mean', except:

   a. It is a measure of central tendency
   b. It is best suited for data with a normal distribution
   c. It is sensitive to extreme values
   d. It is a good summary measure for skewed data
   e. It is a poor summary measure for skewed data

9) Identify the mode from the following set of values: 0, 0, 1, 1, 1, 1, 2, 2, 2, 3, 4, 6, 6, 9.

   a. 0
   b. 1
   c. 2
   d. 3
   e. 6

10) Which of the following is not a measure of dispersion?

a. Range
b. Mid-range
c. Interquartile range
d. Variants
e. Standard deviation

11) Which of the following statements is not true regarding standard deviation?

a. It is a measure of dispersion
b. The square root of variance is standard deviation
c. It is usually represented by σ
d. It is usually represented by σ^2
e. None of the above

12) In a distribution that is skewed to the left, all of the following statements are true, except:

a. Mean, mode and median are on the same line
b. Mean is towards the tail
c. Median is in the middle
d. Mode is towards the right
e. Use of median is preferred to represent the centre of the data

13) Which of the following statements best describes a confidence interval?

a. It helps to calculate the mean
b. It helps to calculate the mode
c. It helps to calculate the median
d. It is the same as interquartile range
e. It indicates how precise or imprecise the estimate is

14) Which of the following measures of central tendency has half of the observations below it and half of the observations above it?

a. Arithmetic mean
b. Geometric mean
c. Median
d. Mode
e. Range

15) Which of the following is the most commonly used measure of central location?

a. Arithmetic mean
b. Geometric mean
c. Median
d. Mode
e. Range

16) All of the following are measures of dispersion, except:

    a. Variance
    b. Standard deviation
    c. Range
    d. Percentile
    e. Interquartile range

17) Which of the following describes the distribution curve below?

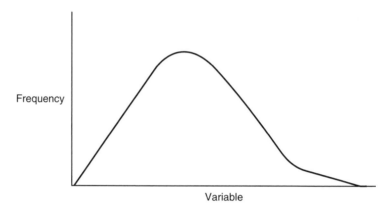

    a. Negatively skewed
    b. Positively skewed
    c. Skewed to the left
    d. Normal distribution
    e. None of the above

18) Which of the following measures of central location is most affected by extreme values?

    a. Range
    b. Mode
    c. Median
    d. Geometric mean
    e. Arithmetic mean

19) Which of the following data sets has the smallest standard deviation?

    a. 2, 4, 4, 4, 6, 9, 9, 9, 10, 10
    b. 6, 8, 8, 8, 11, 12, 13, 14, 15, 16
    c. 1, 1, 1, 6, 6, 6, 6, 6, 6, 6
    d. 2, 4, 6, 8, 10, 12, 14, 16
    e. 30, 30, 30, 30, 30, 30, 30, 30, 30, 30

20) Which of the following is essential for testing the effectiveness of a given treatment?

   a. Untreated controls
   b. Double-blind procedure
   c. A valid measure of change
   d. Patients' self-reports
   e. Physiological measures

21) Which of the following is not typically included in a study protocol?

   a. Aims of the study
   b. Review of relevant literature
   c. Study design
   d. Anticipated date of the start of the study
   e. Anticipated date of the publication of results

22) All of the following are essential qualities of a well designed study, except:

   a. Clearly defined inclusion and exclusion criteria
   b. Power calculation
   c. Use of reliable and valid instruments
   d. Excluding the data from drop-outs to avoid spurious results
   e. Intention-to-treat analysis

23) Placebo-controlled studies are justifiable in which of the following scenarios?

   a. When a new drug is developed
   b. To measure mortality risk
   c. To convince people to use a new drug
   d. When there is no possibility of treatment being better than placebo
   e. When there is genuine uncertainty as to whether the treatment is better than placebo

24) Which of the following statements is true regarding data collection?

   a. Questionnaires sent by mail usually get a response rate of less than 40%
   b. The maximum amount of data should be collected from the records
   c. The General Health Questionnaire (GHQ) can be used to screen for psychosis
   d. The Present State Examination is a structured interview for mental state examination
   e. The Schedule for Affective Disorders and Schizophrenia (SADS) is a structured interview

25) Which of the following statements is true regarding study designs?

    a. Observation studies can be used to establish the direction of causality
    b. Case-control studies give information about prevalence
    c. Case-control studies give information about incidence
    d. Sex cannot be a confounder
    e. Cohort studies provide information about relative risk

26) Which of the following statements is not true regarding research data?

    a. It is conventional to report 90% confidence intervals
    b. In normal distribution, the probability of the population mean lying more than two standard errors away from the sample mean is less than 5%
    c. Confidence intervals can be calculated from the mean and standard error only if the variable is assumed to be normally distributed
    d. The standard error of the mean enables estimation of the range within which the mean would fall if the study were repeated
    e. The standard error of the mean is a function of the standard deviation of the sample and of the sample size

27) Type II error is caused by which of the following?

    a. Non-random recruitment
    b. Too many groups in the study design
    c. Too many subjects
    d. Too few subjects
    e. None of the above

28) Which of the following statements is not true regarding the principles of meta-analysis?

    a. All studies should be given equal weight
    b. Double-blind randomized controlled trials are the gold standard
    c. The topic to be reviewed must be clearly defined
    d. Studies published in a wide range of journals should be included
    e. Publication bias can be reduced by using a funnel plot

29) Which of the following statements is true regarding frequency measures?

    a. Prevalence rates are a measure of new cases
    b. Incidence can be determined by performing a cross-sectional survey
    c. Incidence is a proportion and can therefore be best expressed as a percentage
    d. With prevalence rates, the denominator is a percentile
    e. Chronic diseases have a low incidence and a high prevalence

30) Which of the following statements is not true regarding statistical power?

a. It gives the probability that a type I error will not occur
b. It depends upon the strength of the expected association in relation to the measurement error
c. It depends upon the prevalence of the exposure
d. It depends upon the significance level chosen
e. It depends upon the sample size

31) Which of the following statements is true regarding randomized controlled trials?

a. A double-blind design eliminates the chance of measurement bias
b. They are observational studies
c. They can be thought of as matched cohort studies in which unknown confounders are randomly allocated
d. Subjects who drop out should be left out of the final analysis
e. If the randomization is not biased, it is not necessary to analyse the data for potentially confounding variables

32) All of the following statements are true regarding confounding variables in epidemiological research, except:

a. They can be either a risk factor or a protective factor
b. They can be associated with both exposure and disease
c. They can be taken into account by introducing randomization in a study design
d. They are on the causal pathway between exposure and disease
e. They can be taken into account by introducing matching into a study design

33) In experimental studies, which of the following is not a form of group comparison?

a. Parallel groups
b. Cross-over design
c. Double blinding
d. Factorial design
e. Sequential design

34) Which of the following methods of data collection is the most expensive and time consuming but can generate high-quality data?

a. Computer interview
b. Telephone interview
c. Mail questionnaires
d. Personal interview
e. Record reviews

35) Which of the following statements is not true regarding correlation?

   a. It is a useful technique to analyse nominal data
   b. It usually examines the association between two variables (X and Y)
   c. A 0 correlation means that there is no association between X and Y
   d. A positive correlation means that Y increases in a straight line as X increases
   e. A negative correlation means that Y decreases in a straight line as X increases

36) What is the range of the correlation coefficient?

   a. 0 to +1
   b. −1 to 0
   c. 0 to +100
   d. −100 to 0
   e. −1 to +1

37) Which of the following statements is not true regarding systematic reviews?

   a. They deal with a specific research question
   b. They clearly explain the search strategy
   c. They pool the results from the selected studies
   d. They can be valuable for evidence-based practice
   e. Overall conclusions are not more reliable than individual studies

38) Which of the following could negatively influence the conclusions of a meta-analysis?

   a. Combining the results of several studies
   b. Calculation of a P value from the pooled data
   c. Calculation of a confidence interval from the pooled data
   d. Interpretation of the findings
   e. Publication bias

39) Which of the following statements is not true regarding forest plots?

   a. They are used to present results of randomized controlled trials only
   b. The studies are listed on the vertical axis
   c. The outcome measure is on the horizontal axis
   d. The 'line of unity' intersects the horizontal access
   e. The overall outcome is represented by the diamond shape

40) Which of the following statistical methods is not used to test for heterogeneity?

   a. Forest plot
   b. Galbraith plot
   c. Z statistic
   d. Chi-square statistic
   e. The Peto method

41) Which of the following statements best explains the term 'publication bias'?

a. Studies with negative findings are more likely to be published
b. Studies with positive findings are more likely to be published
c. Studies with high mortality figures are more likely to be published
d. Studies with low mortality figures are more likely to be published
e. Studies sponsored by drug companies are more likely to be published

42) Which of the following methods can be used to identify publication bias?

a. Graphical method
b. Meta regression
c. Correlation coefficient
d. Funnel plots
e. Forest plots

43) Which of the following study designs would be most suitable for aetiological studies?

a. Cross-sectional studies
b. Case-controlled studies
c. Randomized controlled trials
d. Intervention studies
e. None of the above

44) Suppose a test on cerebrospinal fluid has been developed to identify depression. Which of the following terms best explains the following situation: 'A patient has been given a negative result when he is actually suffering from depression'?

a. True positive
b. True negative
c. False negative
d. False positive
e. None of the above

45) Which of the following statements best describes the 'positive predictive value' of a screening test?

a. The proportion of people getting a positive result who will have the disease
b. The proportion of people with the disease who test positive
c. The proportion of people without the disease who test negative
d. The proportion of people getting a negative result who will not have the disease
e. The likelihood that those who test positive will have the disease as opposed to not have the disease

6. Research methods, evidence-based practice, statistics and critical appraisal I: Questions

46) What is the most suitable study design for assessing the effectiveness of a newly developed treatment?

a. Retrospective study
b. Cross-sectional study
c. Randomized controlled trial
d. Observational study
e. Systematic review

47) Which of the following statements best describes the term 'number needed to treat'?

a. The number of patients needed to be treated for the completion of a particular trial
b. The number of patients who must be treated with an intervention without experiencing any adverse side-effects
c. The number of patients who must be treated with a particular intervention for one patient to experience the beneficial effect
d. It means the same as absolute risk reduction
e. It means the same as 'number needed to harm'

48) Which of the following statements is not true regarding survival analysis?

a. It is usually applicable to longitudinal cohort studies
b. It looks exclusively at rate and time of death
c. It can be used to calculate the median survival time
d. It can be used to predict the likelihood of a number of outcomes in the study group
e. It is not useful for cross-sectional studies

49) Which of the following statements best explains the term 'cost-effectiveness analysis'?

a. An analysis of an intervention to cut down a cost
b. An analysis of a number of interventions to cut down the cost
c. An analysis to compare multiple interventions that produce the same beneficial outcome with a similar degree of benefit
d. An analysis of the cost of a number of interventions for achieving a particular desired effect
e. An analysis of multiple interventions to choose the most suitable one for a particular condition

50) Which of the following statements is not true regarding qualitative research?

a. It analyses the quality of data produced by a randomized controlled trial
b. It looks at the subjective experiences of the participants
c. It is useful for investigating attitudes and beliefs of the participants
d. It does not necessarily require a hypothesis at the beginning of the research
e. The stress is on the quality and depth of information gathered during research

6. Research methods, evidence-based practice, statistics and critical appraisal 1: Answers

1) e.
Relative risk compares the risk of some health-related event, such as a disease or death, in two groups. The group of primary interest is labelled the exposed group and the comparison group is labelled the unexposed group. The relative risk is calculated according to the following equation:

$$\text{Relative risk} = \frac{\text{risk of exposed group}}{\text{risk of unexposed group}}$$

A risk ratio of 1.0 indicates identical risks in the two groups. A risk ratio greater than 1.0 indicates an increased risk for the exposed group and a risk ratio less than 1.0 indicates a decreased risk for the exposed group.

2) d.
Odds ratio is a measure of association that qualifies the relationship between an exposure and health outcome for a comparative study. The odds ratio is also sometimes called the cross-product ratio, as it is obtained by the product of the number of diseased people with exposure and the number of healthy people without exposure divided by the product of healthy people with exposure and diseased people without exposure.

3) a.
The placebo drugs, although pharmacologically inert, do produce effects, as reported by the participants of the trial.

4) d.
The placebo effect is least likely to be influenced by the age of the patient.

5) b.
A measure of central location such as arithmetic mean, median or mode is a single value that best represents a particular characteristic such as age or height of a group of individuals.

6) d.
Range is a measure of dispersion.

7) a.
The symmetrical clustering of values around a central location is typical of many frequency distributions and is called the normal distribution. The

bell-shaped curve that results when a normal distribution is crafted is also called the normal curve. The common bell-shaped distribution is the basis of many tests that are used to draw conclusions or make generalizations from the data.

8) d.
Arithmetic mean, because of its sensitivity to extreme values, is considered a poor summary measure for data that are severely skewed in either a positive or a negative direction.

9) b.
Mode is the value that occurs most often in a set of data and in this example the number 1 occurs four times, which is more than any other value.

10) b.
Mid-range is a measure of central tendency.

11) d.
Variance and standard deviation are measures of dispersion. Variance is the mean of the square differences of the observations from the mean. It is usually represented in formulas as σ^2. The standard deviation is the square root of variance and is usually represented in formulas as σ.

12) a.
Mean, mode and median lie on the same line in symmetrical distribution and not in skewed distribution. In skewed distributions, the median is preferred to represent the centre of the data because it is not affected by a few extremely high or low observations.

13) e.
A confidence interval indicates how precise or imprecise an estimate is. A confidence level is usually set at 95%.

14) c.
The median is at the halfway point of a set of data that have been arranged in rank order.

15) a.
The arithmetic mean is the most commonly used measure of central location.

16) d.
A percentile is at a particular point in a data set and is not a measure of dispersion.

17) b.

This distribution curve is positively skewed as the tail points to the right and defines the direction of the skew. A distribution with a tail to the right and a central location to the left is said to be positively skewed or skewed to the right.

18) e.

The arithmetic mean is most sensitive to extreme values.

19) e.

As all the observations have the same value, the mean is 30, the difference between each value and the mean is 0 and thus the standard deviation is also 0. In other words, there is no dispersion from the mean.

20) c.

A validated instrument to measure a change is essential for testing the effectiveness of a given treatment.

21) e.

The anticipated date and place of publication of the results is usually not included in a study protocol.

22) d.

The data from drop-outs should always be included in an intention-to-treat analysis.

23) e.

A placebo-controlled study can be justifiable only if there is genuine uncertainty as to whether the active treatment is better than placebo.

24) d.

The Present State Examination is a structured mental state interview. The response rates to mail questionnaires are usually between 40 and 60%. The GHQ is a screening instrument for non-psychotic illness and the SADS is a semi-structured interview.

25) e.

Cohort studies do provide information about relative risk, which is the ratio of illness rates in the exposed to the unexposed. Observational studies can provide clues only to causality but they cannot establish the direction of causality. Case-control studies give clues to aetiology. Sex can be confounding as it is a variable related to both risk factors and illness.

26) a.

It is conventional to report 95% confidence intervals.

27) d.

With too few subjects there is a high risk of type II error or a false negative result.

28) a.

Larger studies should be given greater weight.

29) e.

Incidence is the rate of new cases occurring in a defined population in a given time period, whereas prevalence is the proportion of a defined population that has the disease at a given time. Chronic diseases tend to show higher prevalence figures than incidence as the patient survives for a longer time and the total number of patients is always higher than the number of new cases.

30) a.

Statistical power gives the probability that a type II error will not occur. The statistical power increases with increases in **b, c, d** and **e**.

31) c.

Blinding can only reduce the chance of measurement bias but cannot eliminate it. Randomized controlled trials are not observational studies but experimental studies. Drop-outs have to be considered in an intention-to-treat analysis. It is important to analyse data for potentially confounding variables as even unbiased randomization can result in differences between the groups.

32) d.

The confounding variables are not on the causal pathway between exposure and disease.

33) c.

Double blinding is not a form of group comparison but a technique used in randomized controlled trials where the researcher and the subject are blinded from the information about whether the subject is entering the treatment arm or placebo arm of the study. Double blinding helps to prevent observation bias as well as placebo effect.

34) d.

The personal interview approach can generate high-quality data with a high response rate but is expensive and time consuming. It also requires training and practice for the interviewers.

35) a.

Correlation is used to look at the association between continuous quantitative data.

36) e.
The correlation coefficient ranges from -1 to $+1$. It is used in research to show the strength of the linear relationship between two variables.

37) e.
Systematic reviews are considered the gold-standard source for research evidence and overall conclusions are usually more reliable than those drawn from individual studies.

38) e.
Publication bias can have a negative effect on the findings of a meta-analysis. Ideally, a meta-analysis should include all the information provided by all the studies performed to answer a particular question. If the results of only positive studies are considered for meta-analysis, then the findings could be biased towards a particular intervention, as all the negative studies were excluded.

39) a.
Forest plots are generally used to present the results of a meta-analysis.

40) e.
The Peto method is used for individual and combined odds ratios.

41) b.
Publication bias means the studies with positive findings are more likely to be published.

42) d.
Funnel plots are used to identify publication bias. If publication bias is absent, then the funnel plot is symmetrical; it becomes asymmetrical in the presence of publication bias.

43) b.
In case-controlled studies, patients with a particular disease are identified and their past exposure to the aetiological factors is studied and compared with that of control subjects who do not have the disease. The odds ratio is estimated and potential confounding factors are measured.

44) c.
A false-negative result means that a negative result has been shown by the test when the patient is actually suffering from depression.

45) a.
The positive predictive value is the proportion of people scoring positive on the test who will have the disease.

46) c.

Randomized controlled trials are considered the gold standard for assessing the effectiveness of a newly developed intervention.

47) c.

The number needed to treat is the number of patients who must be treated with an intervention for one patient to experience the benefit of the treatment.

48) b.

Survival analysis is not exclusively used for information on time to death but can be applied to a number of outcomes.

49) d.

Cost-effectiveness analysis is an economic analysis aiming to compare the cost of multiple interventions that achieve the same effect.

50) a.

Qualitative research collects and analyses data that cannot be presented as numbers; it is used in the initial stages of research, studies dealing with attitudes and beliefs, assessment tools development, etc.

Further reading

Actuarial Science Department at Simon Fraser University. Available at: www.stat.sfu.ca.

Gelder M, Harrison P, Cowen P. *Shorter Oxford Textbook of Psychiatry*, 5th edn. Oxford: Oxford University Press, 2006.

Gosall N, Gosall G. *The Doctor's Guide to Critical Appraisal*. Knutsford, Cheshire: PasTest, 2006.

Greenhalgh T. *How to Read a Paper: The Basics of Evidence-Based Medicine*, 2nd edn. London: BMJ, 2001.

Lawry S, McIntosh A, Rao S. *Critical Appraisal for Psychiatrists*. Edinburgh: Churchill Livingstone, 2000.

Puri B, Hall A. *Revision Notes in Psychiatry*, 2nd edn. London: Arnold/Hodder Education, 2004.

7. Research methods, evidence-based practice, statistics and critical appraisal 2: Questions

1) Which of the following statements is not correct regarding the principles of causal inference?

   a. Lack of temporal ambiguity means that the cause should precede the effect
   b. A dose–response relationship means that the size of an effect should vary with the size of the cause
   c. Coherence means that there is no biological or theoretical basis for the hypothesized cause and effect
   d. Specificity means that the effects are associated primarily with one cause
   e. Consistency means that the same relationship is seen over many studies involving a wide range of other factors

2) The height in centimetres of five medical students is 165, 175, 176, 159 and 170. Which of the following pairs are the median and mean of the sample?

   a. 170, 169
   b. 170, 170
   c. 169, 170
   d. 176, 169
   e. 176, 176

3) The depression scores on the Hamilton Anxiety and Depression Scale administered to a group of 11 patients are as follows:

   16, 18, 20, 20, 22, 24, 26, 26, 26, 28, 30.

   Which of the following pairs are the median and mode of the sample?

   a. 26, 20
   b. 24, 20
   c. 24, 26
   d. 16, 30
   e. 22, 26

4) In a large data set looking at the age of onset of schizophrenia in males, if the majority of ages are similar (18–20 years) but a few findings showing a very high age of around 50 years, how would the mean and median of these data compare and what would be the shape of the histogram?

a. The mean would be smaller than the median and the histogram would be skewed with a long left tail
b. The mean would be larger than the median and the histogram would be skewed with a long right tail
c. The mean would be larger than the median and the histogram would be skewed with a long left tail
d. The mean would be smaller than the median and the histogram would be skewed with a long right tail
e. The mean would be equal to the median and the histogram would be symmetrical

5) In skewed distributions, the median is preferred over the mean for most purposes because:

a. The median is the most frequent number while the mean is most likely
b. The mean may be too heavily influenced by a few extreme observations
c. The median is less than the mean and smaller numbers are always appropriate for the centre
d. The mean measures the spread in the data
e. The median measures the arithmetic average of the data excluding outliers

6) Which of the following statements would in general be false?

a. The sample mean is more sensitive to extreme values than the median
b. The standard deviation is a measure of spread around the mean
c. The range is more sensitive to extreme values than the standard deviation
d. If a distribution is symmetrical then the mean will be equal to the median
e. The standard deviation is a measure of central tendency around the median

7) The scores of 15 candidates taking an objective structured clinical examination (OSCE) are recorded by the examiners in ascending order as follows:

4, 7, 7, 9, 10, 11, 13, 15, 15, 15, 17, 17, 19, 19, 20.

After calculating the mean, mode and median, an error is discovered by one of the examiners. One of the students, by mistake, has been given 15 instead of 17. Which of the three measures of central tendency (mean, mode and median) already calculated will have to be changed?

a. Mean
b. Mode
c. Median
d. Mean and mode
e. All three

8) Which of the following statements is incorrect?

a. In a symmetrical distribution, the mean and median are equal
b. The first quartile is equal to the 25th percentile
c. In asymmetric distribution, the median is halfway between the first and third quartile
d. The median is always greater than the mean
e. The range is the difference between the largest and the smallest observation in the data set

9) Regarding standard deviation, which of the following statements is false?

a. A data set with values 3, 3 and 3 has a standard deviation of 0
b. A data set with values 3, 4 and 5 has the same standard deviation as a data set with values 103, 104 and 105
c. The standard deviation is a measure of scatter around the centre of the data
d. A data set with values 1, 5 and 9 has a smaller standard deviation than a data set with values 101, 105 and 109
e. The standard deviation is the square root of variance

10) Suppose you are working on a paediatric intensive care unit (PICU) ward and have been told that the chance of physical aggression by the patients is one in every three doctor–patient contacts. During the last nine days you have had one contact with a patient every day and have not had any episode of physical aggression. Today, the 10th day, you are going to interview a patient. What are the chances of physical aggression towards you?

a. Greater than one in three because you have not had any episodes in the last nine days

b. Less than one in three because you have not had any episodes in the last nine days

c. Still equal to one in three because the last nine days do not affect the probability

d. Equal to one in ten because you have not had any episodes in the last nine days

e. Equal to nine in ten because you have not had any episodes in the last nine days

11) Suppose the chance of patients developing depression after the diagnosis of Alzheimer's disease has been estimated to be 1 in 4. What does this mean?

a. Every fourth patient will develop depression after being given the diagnosis of Alzheimer's disease in your clinic

b. Of 1000 people diagnosed with Alzheimer's disease, exactly 250 will become depressed

c. Of 200 people diagnosed with Alzheimer's disease, about 50 will become depressed

d. In exactly 25% of all patients diagnosed with Alzheimer's disease, depression will occur

e. Out of 20 people diagnosed with Alzheimer's disease, it is very likely that exactly five people will become depressed

12) An epidemiological study finds that about 20% of people between the ages of 18 and 25 have smoked cannabis over the last year. Which of the following statements is true in the light of this finding?

a. If five people of this age are randomly selected, one of them must have smoked cannabis in the last year

b. If 20 people are randomly selected from this age group and 18 of them have smoked cannabis in the last year, the 19th person selected at random will have a lower probability of having smoked cannabis

c. If 10 people are randomly selected from this age group and none of them have smoked cannabis over the last year, the next person selected will have a higher probability of having smoked cannabis in the last year

d. If 1000 people from this age group are randomly selected, it will not be unusual to find that around 200 of them have smoked cannabis in the last year

e. If 1 000 000 people from this age group are randomly selected there must be exactly 200 000 of them who have smoked cannabis in the last year

13) Suppose the results of last year's MRCPsych examination paper 1 show that the marks obtained by candidates followed a normal distribution with a mean of 65 and a standard deviation of 12. With the pass mark being 50, approximately what percentage of candidates have failed that examination?

a. 11%
b. 22%
c. 41%
d. 60%
e. 89%

14) A research team looking at use of recreational drugs by teenagers has decided to replicate a study they carried out a few years previously. The statistician advising the team has suggested increasing the size of the random sample of teenagers from 1500 to 4000. What is the likely effect of this increase in the size of sample?

a. A reduction in the bias of the estimate
b. An increase in the standard error of the estimate
c. A reduction in the variability of the findings
d. An increase in the chances of finding higher rates of drug use
e. It will have no effect because the population size is the same

15) Which of the following statements is not true regarding the sampling distribution of the mean?

a. The standard error of the mean is a measure of the variability of the mean among repeated samples
b. The sampling distribution shows how the sample was distributed around the mean
c. The standard error of the mean will decrease as the sample size increases
d. The sampling distribution shows how the mean will vary among repeated samples
e. The mean is unbiased for the true (unknown population) mean

16) Which of the following statements explains best the meaning of 'the sample mean is an unbiased estimator of the population mean'?

a. The sample mean is always very close to the population mean
b. The sample mean is always equal to the population mean
c. The sample mean will vary only a little from the population mean
d. The sample mean has a normal distribution
e. The average sample mean, over all possible samples, equals the population mean

17) Which of the following statements is not true regarding sampling in an epidemiological survey?

a. If proper random sampling procedures are followed, every subject of the population has an equal chance of being selected
b. The precision of the sample mean depends upon the sample size and not on the population size if proper random sampling procedures are followed
c. The sampling distribution of the sample mean describes how the sample mean will vary among repeated samples
d. Convenience sampling often leads to bias because the sample is often not representative of the population
e. If a sample of 1000 families is randomly selected from a town with a total of 10 000 families, and the average family income from the sample is £50, then the true value of the family income for all the families in the town is known

18) A group of researchers decide to look at the possibility of mild to moderate depression in a group of elderly people attending a day hospital. They take a random sample of the subjects to administer a semi-structured interview for the diagnosis of depression. Which of the following statements is not true?

a. A convenience sample could be chosen by selecting the first 25 people entering the day hospital on that particular day
b. The subjects were selected randomly and this means that every person attending the day hospital on the particular day had an equal chance of being selected
c. The confidence interval calculated from the data refers to the proportion of subjects in the sample who were suffering from mild to moderate depression
d. If another sample of subjects is selected, it is likely that a slightly different proportion of subjects with mild to moderate depression will be found
e. Even though the subjects were selected randomly, the sample may not be representative of the elderly people living in the community

19) In a study of the proportion of inpatients on psychiatric units who are suicidal, which of the following statements is not true?

a. Different researchers may get different values for the proportion of inpatients with suicidal ideas
b. If the rules of random sampling are followed, the proportion of inpatients with suicidal ideas found from the study is an unbiased estimate of suicidal ideas in the total inpatient population
c. A convenience sample of the first 20 inpatients may give a biased estimate of the proportion of patients with suicidal ideas
d. A convenience sample of 100 inpatients is always better than a properly drawn random sample of 20 patients
e. A random sample of 100 inpatients will give a more precise estimate of the proportion of patients with suicidal ideas than a sample of 20 inpatients

20) Which of the following statements is not true regarding sampling?

   a. A large sample size always gives unbiased results, regardless of how the sample is selected
   b. The standard error measures how much the answer (outcome) may vary if a new sample of the same size is chosen using the same sampling method
   c. The sampling distribution describes how the answer will vary if a new sample is taken
   d. A randomly chosen larger sample will give answers that vary less from the true value than a randomly chosen smaller sample
   e. The standard deviation measures the variability of the values in a sample

21) Which of the following statements best describes the 'null hypothesis'?

   a. It is the same as the primary hypothesis in a research protocol
   b. It states that any difference observed in the results of the study groups is not due to chance
   c. It states that any difference observed in the results between the groups is due to chance
   d. A properly conducted study will always prove the null hypothesis to be incorrect
   e. A properly conducted study will always prove that the null hypothesis is correct

22) Generally, which of the following P values is accepted as a threshold for statistical significance?

   a. Less than 0.10
   b. Less than 0.09
   c. Less than 0.07
   d. Less than 0.05
   e. Less than 0.01

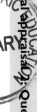

23) What does a P value of less than 0.05 mean?

   a. The probability of obtaining a given result by chance is less than 1 in 5
   b. The probability of obtaining a given result by chance is less than 1 in 10
   c. The probability of obtaining a given result by chance is less than 1 in 20
   d. The probability of obtaining a given result is less than 1 in 50
   e. None of the above

24) In a research paper on the effectiveness of a new antidepressant in the treatment of severe depression, the P value for the subjects on the active drug is 0.10. Which of the following statements is not true?

   a. The results are not significant
   b. The association between the use of the new drug and improvement in mood cannot be proved
   c. The probability of seeing an improvement in mood by chance is high
   d. Null hypothesis is rejected
   e. The P value is higher than the threshold of statistical significance

25) Which of the following statements is not true regarding type I errors?

    a. They are a false positive result
    b. They can be caused by bias
    c. They can be caused by confounding factors
    d. They occur when a true null hypothesis is rejected on the basis of results
    e. They occur when a true null hypothesis is accepted on the basis of results

26) Suppose you have read a research paper on the use of a new antipsychotic. The results reveal that the group of patients treated by the new antipsychotic showed a statistically significant improvement in symptoms, with a P value of 0.05. What are the chances that a type I error occurred, or in other words an erroneous rejection of the null hypothesis?

    a. 5%
    b. 20%
    c. 50%
    d. 0.5%
    e. 0.05%

27) Which of the following statements is not true regarding type II errors?

    a. They are a false negative result
    b. The null hypothesis is accepted when it is actually false
    c. They can be avoided by doing a power calculation
    d. The sample size is too large
    e. The sample size is not large enough

28) Which of the following statements best describes the 'power' of a study?

    a. It increases the impact of the results of the study
    b. It gives the probability that a type I error will not be made
    c. It gives the probability that a type II error will not be made
    d. It should be calculated at the time of the data analysis of a study
    e. It does not have any impact on the number of subjects recruited for a study

29) While planning a study, you consult a statistician colleague, who advises that the power of the study should be 0.8. What does this mean?

    a. 8% probability of finding a statistically significant difference if it exists
    b. 10% probability of finding a statistically significant difference if it exists
    c. 20% probability of finding a statistically significant difference if it exists
    d. 80% probability of finding a statistically significant difference if it exists
    e. 0.8% probability of finding a statistically significant difference if it exists

30) All of the following statistical tests can be used for data that are not normally distributed, except:

a. Fisher's test
b. Wilcoxon rank-sum test
c. Mann–Whitney U test
d. Kruskal–Wallis test
e. Friedman test

31) Which of the following statements is incorrect regarding parametric and non-parametric tests?

a. Parametric tests are used for normally distributed data
b. Non-parametric tests are used for non-normally distributed data
c. A t-test is a parametric test
d. Analysis of variance (ANOVA) is a non-parametric test
e. The Mann–Whitney U test is a non-parametric test

32) Statistical significance can be measured by all of the following tests, except:

a. Probability tests
b. Validity tests
c. t-test
d. Chi-square test
e. ANOVA

33) Which of the following statistical tests is not used in the comparison of data from two or more groups?

a. McNemar's test
b. Fisher's test
c. Mann–Whitney U test
d. Friedman test
e. Kruskal–Wallis ANOVA

34) Which of the following statistical tests would be suitable for comparing more than two groups if the data are non-parametric?

a. Chi-square test
b. Wilcoxon signed rank test
c. Wilcoxon rank-sum test
d. t-test
e. Friedman test

35) Which of the following statements is incorrect regarding hypothesis testing?

a. The power of a study refers to the probability that a type I error will not be made
b. The larger the study sample, the higher is its power for detecting a true difference between two groups
c. Failure to reject a false null hypothesis is called a type II error
d. Falsely rejecting a true null hypothesis is called a type I error
e. The null hypothesis is generally rejected if the P value is less than 0.05

36) Which of the following statements is true regarding the *t*-test?

a. It is a non-parametric test
b. It can be used both on one sample and in comparison of two groups
c. It is used for data which are not normally distributed
d. If it is used for comparing two groups, they have to be of equal size
e. It can be used for positively skewed data

37) Which of the following statements best describes a normal distribution curve?

a. The tail is to the left
b. The tail is to the right
c. The mean always lies to the left of the mode
d. The median, mode and arithmetic mean coincide
e. The normal distribution curves from different data have different shapes and characteristics

38) Which of the following statements is true regarding standard deviation?

a. It is an index of the reliability of the mean
b. It is generally smaller than the standard error of the mean
c. One of its advantages is that it can be manipulated mathematically
d. The standard deviation can be a negative value
e. It is equal to the sum of the differences between all the values and the mean

39) There is a positive association between the number of suicides and the prescription of antidepressant medication. This is an example of an association likely to be caused by which of the following?

a. A common cause
b. Confounding factor
c. Cause and effect relationship
d. Coincidence
e. None of the above

40) A newly developed antidepressant is given to a group of 25 patients suffering from depression. Five days after taking the new antidepressant, 20 of the subjects report marked improvements in their mood. Which of the following conclusions can be reached from this information?

a. The new antidepressant is effective for the treatment of depression
b. Nothing, because the sample size was too small
c. Nothing, because there was no control group for comparison
d. The new antidepressant is better than the old ones
e. The new antidepressant is not effective for the treatment of depression

41) A drug company wants to investigate if a newly developed antipsychotic is effective in reducing the length and severity of psychosis. They recruit the first 20 patients attending a GP surgery with psychotic symptoms. The participants are administered a structured interview to confirm the diagnosis. The patients are prescribed the newly developed antipsychotic and are informed about its effects and side-effects. After 4 weeks, the patients are assessed again, and 15 patients out of the 20 report a reduction in the severity of psychotic symptoms, which is confirmed by administering a structured interview. Which of the following statements is not true about this study?

a. This is not a well designed study as there was no control group. We do not know how many patients would feel better in 4 weeks without treatment
b. This is not a well designed study as it was not double blinded. The patients might have felt better because they thought the drug should work
c. This is not a well designed study because a convenience sample was selected. Patients who come to the GP surgery with psychotic symptoms may have more severe symptoms than people who do not come to the surgery
d. This is not a well designed study because the new antipsychotic was not given to people without psychotic symptoms to assess its effect in a control group
e. This is not a well designed study because the sample size is likely to be too small to detect anything but a change in symptoms in a small group of patients

42) Regarding sampling, which of the following statements is true?

a. In random samples, the randomization ensures that precise and accurate estimates are obtained
b. In a properly chosen sample, an estimate will be less variable with a large sample size and hence more precise
c. If all of the things are equal, a large sample size is needed for a larger population
d. A large sample size always ensures that the sample is representative of the population
e. It is not necessary to randomize if the sample size is sufficiently large

43) A properly conducted random survey selects 1000 Asians (from a population of 10 million) and 1000 Caucasians (from a total population of 100 million). Which of the following statements is not true?

a. Randomization ensures that both samples are representative of their respective populations
b. The precision is determined by the ratio of the sample size to the total population size
c. A smaller proportion of the Caucasian population has been chosen. Therefore, a particular person has a smaller chance of being selected from the Caucasian population as compared with the Asian population
d. The samples are likely to be representative of their respective populations
e. None of the above

44) A team of epidemiologists decides to conduct a survey on the contribution of the mental health services to the NHS. A questionnaire is circulated to 100 academics whom the team decides 'are the most likely to know how important mental health services are for the NHS'. Which of the following is the main problem with using data from this survey to draw conclusions?

a. Interviewer bias
b. Non-response bias
c. No control group
d. Insufficient attention to the placebo effect
e. Selection bias

45) While administering a depression questionnaire to a patient in accident and emergency, the duty doctor notices that the patient has scored high on risk of suicide. If the patient is admitted, he will take up the only bed left on the ward. If the patient is not admitted, then he may commit suicide. In this situation what would be the appropriate null hypothesis and a type I error?

a. Null hypothesis is assuming that the suicidal warning can be ignored. Type I error is deciding to admit the patient when the patient is not suicidal
b. Null hypothesis is assuming the suicide warning can be ignored. Type I error is deciding not to admit the patient when the patient is suicidal
c. Null hypothesis is assuming that all patients scoring high on the questionnaire should be admitted. Type I error is deciding to ignore the warning when the patient is suicidal
d. Null hypothesis is assuming that all patients scoring high on the questionnaire should be admitted. Type I error is deciding to admit the patient when the patient is not suicidal
e. Null hypothesis is assuming that all that depressed patients should be admitted. Type I error is demanding unlimited beds for depressed patients coming to A&E

46) Which of the following statements is not true?

a. The P value measures the probability that the null hypothesis is true
b. The power of a test depends upon the sample size and the distance between the null and alternative hypotheses
c. A probability of a type II error is controlled by the sample size
d. The probability of a type I error is controlled by the selection of the alpha level
e. The rejection region is controlled by the alpha level and the alternative hypothesis

47) A research study on treatment of Alzheimer's disease is carried out on a random sample of 30 patients. On data analysis, a test of significance is conducted under appropriate null and alternative hypotheses and the P value is calculated to be 0.03. What does this result mean?

a. This result is statistically significant at the 0.01 level
b. The probability of being wrong in this situation is only 0.03
c. There is some reason to believe that the null hypothesis is incorrect
d. If the study were repeated, 3% of the time the same result would be obtained
e. The sample is so small that little confidence can be placed on the result

48) Which of the following statements is true regarding the P value?

    a. An extremely small P value indicates that the actual data differ markedly from that expected if the null hypothesis were true

    b. The P value measures the probability that the hypothesis is true

    c. The P value measures the probability of making a type II error

    d. The larger the P value, the stronger is the evidence against the null hypothesis

    e. A large P value indicates that the data are inconsistent with the alternative hypothesis

49) A study is carried out to investigate the effectiveness of a new anxiolytic drug. 1000 subjects participate in the study, with 500 being randomly assigned to the treatment group and the other 500 to the control group. A statistically significant difference with a P value of 0.005 is reported between the responses of the two groups. Which of the following statements best explains the results of the study?

    a. There is evidence of a strong treatment effect

    b. There is little evidence that the treatment has any effect

    c. There is strong evidence that there is some difference in effect between the treatment and the placebo

    d. There is strong evidence that the treatment is very effective

    e. There is a large difference between the effects of treatment and placebo

50) You are planning to conduct a trial to compare two antidepressants: a newly developed one with an old one. You want to see whether there is sufficient evidence to say that the new antidepressant is better than the old one. While conducting the trial you will commit a type I error if:

    a. You conclude that the drugs are equal in effectiveness when in fact the new drug is better

    b. You conclude that the drugs are equal in effectiveness when in fact the old drug is better

    c. You conclude that the old drug is better when in fact the new drug is better

    d. You conclude that the new drug is better when in fact the drugs are equal in effectiveness

    e. You conclude that the old drug is better when in fact the drugs are equal in effectiveness

51) In a study plan to investigate the efficacy of different antidepressant medications, which of the following statements is the best argument for assigning the treatment randomly between different groups?

a. Randomization makes the trial easy to conduct
b. Randomization tends to average out the uncontrolled factors that may confound the treatment effect
c. Randomization makes the data analysis easier
d. Randomization is a requirement for statisticians before starting a trial
e. Randomization means that it is not necessary to be careful when assigning treatment groups

52) Suppose that in 1990 a smoking survey on 350 adult females revealed that 148 smoked and that in 2000 a similar survey on 488 adult females showed that 163 smoked. From an analysis comparing the two results, the P value was found to be 0.053. Which of the following statements best describes this result?

a. The probability that the proportion of smokers has not changed is 0.053
b. The proportion of smokers has definitely decreased
c. There is some, but not overwhelming, evidence that the proportion of smokers has decreased
d. There is no evidence that the proportion of smokers is the same in both years
e. There is overwhelming evidence that the proportion of smokers has stayed the same

53) When using the analysis of variance technique, which of the following is not a necessary assumption?

a. The samples are independent and randomly selected
b. The populations are normally distributed
c. The variances of populations are the same
d. The means of the populations are the same
e. All of the above

54) A research study has reported that there is a correlation of $R = -0.57$ between the hair colour (black, blonde, red) of people and the amount of alcohol that is fatal when consumed. What is the best possible explanation?

a. The lethal dose of alcohol goes down as the hair colour changes
b. Alcohol is less harmful to one hair colour than the other
c. Doctors must always consider hair colour while treating patients with alcohol overdose
d. The researchers of the study need to further explain the causes of this negative correlation
e. The researchers need to take a course in statistics because correlation is not an appropriate measure of association in this situation

55) The summary of an epidemiological study states the following: 'There is a high and positive correlation between body weight and annual income.' Which of the following best explains this statement?

a. High income causes people to gain weight
b. People with high income tend to spend a bigger proportion of their income on food than people with low income, on average
c. Low income leads people to eat less food
d. People with higher income tend to be heavier than people with low income, on average
e. High income causes people to eat more food

56) You have been asked to review the findings of a study that has reported a correlation of $R = -0.45$ between gender (male or female) and income. Which of the following statements is most likely to be your response?

a. The statistician has got it totally wrong
b. There has been an error as R cannot be negative in this scenario
c. On average, women earn more than men
d. On average, women earn less than men
e. None of the above

57) Which of the following statements best defines correlation coefficient?

a. It measures the strength of the linear association between two quantitative variables
b. It measures the strength of the linear association between two categorical variables
c. It measures the extent to which changes in one variable cause changes in another variable
d. It is a measure of the strength of association between two categorical variables
e. It is a measure of the strength of the linear association between a quantitative variable and a categorical variable

58) A study of blood pressure variations in depressed patients randomly selects 20 inpatients and records their blood pressures in the morning and at bedtime. It then looks at the correlation between the morning and night-time blood pressure recordings. What might be the most appropriate expectation?

a. Correlation to be near 0 as the morning and night-time readings should be independent of one another
b. Correlation to be high and positive as those patients with a high reading in the morning will tend to have a higher reading in the evening
c. Correlation to be high and negative as those with a high reading in the morning will tend to have a low reading in the evening
d. Correlation to be near 0 as correlation measures the strength of linear association
e. Correlation to be near 0 as blood-pressure reading should follow approximately a normal distribution

59) In a study on gender and colour preference, each participant (male or female) in a random sample is asked to state his or her preferred colour out of red, blue and green. The following frequencies are reported.

Sex	Red	Green	Blue
Men	3	6	11
Women	17	2	11

Which of the following statements is not true regarding these data?

a. About 15% of the participants are male
b. About 55% of males prefer blue
c. Of those participants who prefer green, about 75% are males
d. A lower percentage of females prefer blue than do males
e. A higher percentage of females prefer red

60) Which of the following would be classified as quantitative data?

a. Nominal data
b. Ordinal data
c. Binary data
d. Multicategory data
e. Discrete numerical data

61) On looking at a data set, you see the body-temperature recordings of all the inpatients on a psychiatric unit. What type of data are these?

a. Nominal data
b. Discrete numerical data
c. Continuous numerical data
d. Categorical data
e. Binary categorical data

62) Which of the following statements best defines the term 'standard error'?

a. The expected statistical error while calculating the mean
b. The error in the sample mean
c. Another name for confidence interval
d. The standard deviation of the sample mean
e. None of the above

63) Which of the following statements is not true regarding confidence intervals?

a. They express the degree of uncertainty around a particular estimate
b. The width of confidence interval indicates the precision of the estimate
c. The greater the width of the confidence interval, the more confidence one can have about the accuracy
d. 95% confidence intervals are routinely reported
e. The larger the sample size, the narrower is the confidence interval

64) Which of the following statements best describes the alternative hypothesis?

a. It is the same as null hypothesis
b. It states that any difference observed between the groups is due to chance
c. It states that the difference observed between the groups is not due to chance
d. If the alternative hypothesis is accepted, then it does not reject the null hypothesis
e. A statistically significant result for differences between groups rejects the alternative hypothesis

65) Which of the following statements is not true regarding a statistically significant result?

a. Null hypothesis is rejected
b. Alternative hypothesis is accepted
c. P value is less than 0.05
d. It is the same as clinical significance
e. It might not be clinically useful

7. Research methods, evidence-based practice, statistics and critical appraisal 2: Answers

1) c.

Coherence means that there is a theoretical, factual, biological and statistical basis for the proposed theory of cause and effect. An example of biological coherence could be the hypothesis stating that hepatitis B infection is the cause of liver cancer. This hypothesis is supported by the finding that the presence of the serological marker of hepatitis B infection is associated with greatly elevated rates of liver cancer and the detection of the viral genome in many liver cancers.

2) a.

Median is the middle value and 170 is the middle value of the five values given. The mean of the sample is the arithmetic mean and is calculated by adding the five values and dividing them by five: $165 + 175 + 176 + 159 + 170 = 845$; $845/5 = 169$.

3) c.

Median is the central value in the sample, which is 24, and mode is the most frequently occurring value in the sample, which is 26.

4) b.

The mean would be larger than the median as the arithmetic mean is very sensitive to extreme values and the median represents the central value. The histogram would be skewed to the right with a long tail due to a few cases developing schizophrenia at the late age of around 50 years.

5) b.

In skewed distributions, a small number of extreme values can have a major effect on the mean, hence the preference for median.

6) e.

The standard deviation is not a measure of central tendency but a measure of dispersion.

7) d.

The mean and mode will change but the median will stay the same.

8) d.

The median is not always greater than the mean, as the mean is sensitive to extreme values and can change with the changes in the data set.

9) d.
A data set with values 1, 5 and 9 will have the same standard deviation as a data set with values 101, 105 and 109.

10) c.
The probability of physical aggression remains the same and is not affected by the events of the last nine days.

11) c.
A 1 in 4 chance of developing depression after diagnosis of Alzheimer's disease means that about 50 in 200 will develop depression.

12) d.
The 20% figure means that about 200 young people in a random sample of 1000 are likely to have smoked cannabis over the last 12 months.

13) a.
If the mean score of candidates was 65 with a standard deviation of 12 then the proportion of candidates with scores below 50 is going to be around 11%.

14) c.
The increase in random sample size is likely to reduce the variability of the findings regarding use of recreational drugs by teenagers.

15) d.
The sampling distribution shows how the mean was distributed in a particular sample.

16) e.
The average sample mean, over all possible samples, equals the population mean.

17) e.
The average family income calculated from the sample cannot provide the true value of the family income for all the families in the town. It provides only the average family income, which will vary from one individual family to another in the town.

18) c.
The confidence interval calculated refers to the likelihood of the mean depression score calculated from the sample being close to the true mean.

19) d.
A smaller but properly drawn random sample is better than a bigger convenience sample.

20) a.
A large sample size does not necessarily give unbiased results if the sample is not chosen randomly.

21) c.
The null hypothesis assumes that any differences observed between the groups are due to chance. If the results show that the differences between the groups cannot be explained by chance alone, then the null hypothesis is rejected.

22) d.
A P value of less than 0.05 is generally accepted as a threshold for statistical significance.

23) c.
A P value of less than 0.05 means that the probability of obtaining a given result by chance is less than 1 in 20.

24) d.
In this case the null hypothesis is accepted, as the results are more likely to be explained by chance alone.

25) e.
A type I error occurs when the null hypothesis is rejected on the basis of results when it is actually true.

26) a.
The probability of making a type I error is equal to the P value; in this particular example, a P value of 0.05 means that there is only a 5% chance of a false positive result or a type I error.

27) d.
Type II errors occur when, due to a small sample size, a study fails to uncover a difference between the groups that actually exists.

28) c.
The power of a study gives the probability that a type II error will not be made and ensures that the study sample is large enough to detect a statistically significant result.

29) d.
A power of 0.8 means that there is an 80% probability of getting a statistically significant difference with a particular sample size if a real difference does exist.

30) a.
Fisher's test is used for normally distributed data.

31) d.
Analysis of variance (ANOVA) is used for parametric data.

32) b.
Validity tests are used to measure the validity of a particular instrument. They do not measure statistical significance.

33) b.
Fisher's test is not used to compare data from two or more groups.

34) e.
The Friedman test would be most suitable to compare non-parametric data for more than two groups.

35) a.
The power of a study refers to the probability that a type II error will not be made

36) b.
A *t*-test is used for normally distributed parametric data.

37) d.
In a normal distribution curve, the median, mode and arithmetic mean coincide.

38) c.
One of the advantages of the standard deviation is that it can be manipulated mathematically.

39) a.
A positive association between suicide and prescription of antidepressants is likely to be due to a common cause (depression).

40) c.
From the given information we cannot reach any conclusion about the effectiveness of the newly developed antidepressant as there was no control group for comparison.

41) d.

Giving the newly developed antipsychotic to people without symptoms is not necessary to assess its antipsychotic properties.

42) b.

In a properly chosen sample, a large sample size ensures less variability of an estimate.

43) b.

The precision is determined mainly by the sample size and not the ratio of the sample size to the total population.

44) e.

Selection bias is the main problem here, as the respondents have not been chosen randomly.

45) a.

We would treat the high suicidal score on the questionnaire as data. The null hypothesis would be that this high suicidal score is not true and can be ignored. Type I error would be to admit the patient if he scores high on the questionnaire when he is not suicidal.

46) a.

The null hypothesis assumes that the findings were due to chance and the P value measures the probability that the findings were not due to chance, or in other words 'the null hypothesis is not true'.

47) c.

In this very small study, although the P value is statistically significant (<0.05), it is safe to conclude that there is some evidence to suggest that the null hypothesis is incorrect.

48) a.

If the P value is extremely small, then it indicates that the actual data differ significantly from the result expected if the null hypothesis were true.

49) c.

The very low P value in this study gives strong evidence that there is some difference in effect between the treatment and placebo. The effectiveness of treatment is different from statistical significance. A difference between two groups that is statistically significant might have no practical importance.

50) d.

A type I error (false positive) would be committed if you concluded that the new drug is better when in fact both drugs are equally effective.

51) b.

Randomization averages out the uncontrolled factors that might act as confounders.

52) c.

The study looking at a possible reduction in the proportion of smokers has revealed a P value of 0.053, which shows that there is some evidence of a decrease in the proportion of smokers.

53) d.

While using ANOVA we cannot assume that the means of the populations are the same.

54) e.

Correlation is not an appropriate measure in this situation as it cannot be computed with nominal variables.

55) d.

We cannot make any causal connections between income and weight gain from these findings; the only plausible inference would be that, on average, people with higher income tend to be heavier than people with low income.

56) a.

Correlation is not an appropriate measure of association in this scenario.

57) a.

The correlation coefficient is defined as a measure of the strength of the linear association between two quantitative variables.

58) b.

As hypertension presents with constantly elevated blood pressure readings then the reasonable expectation would be a high and positive correlation between the morning and evening recordings. Those patients with high readings in the morning will tend to have a higher reading in the evening.

59) a.

A total of 20 males and 30 females participated in the study, which brings the male participant percentage to 40%.

60) e.

Quantitative data are numerical and can be subdivided into discrete numerical data and continuous numerical data.

61) c.

Body temperatures are continuous numerical data as they can be measured; they are a subtype of quantitative data.

62) d.

The standard deviation of the sample means is known as the standard error and is calculated by the following equation: standard error (sample size, n) = standard deviation divided by square root of n.

63) c.

The confidence in making inferences about the population increases as the confidence interval becomes narrower.

64) c.

The alternative hypothesis states that the differences observed between the groups is not due to chance.

65) d.

Statistical significance is not the same as clinical significance, as a statistically significant result might not be meaningful or practically useful in everyday clinical practice.

Further reading

Actuarial Science Department at Simon Fraser University. Available at: www.stat.sfu.ca.

Gelder M, Harrison P, Cowen P. *Shorter Oxford Textbook of Psychiatry*, 5th edn. Oxford: Oxford University Press, 2006.

Gosall N, Gosall G. *The Doctor's Guide to Critical Appraisal*. Knutsford, Cheshire: PasTest, 2006.

Greenhalgh T. *How to Read a Paper: The Basics of Evidence-Based Medicine*, 2nd edn. London: BMJ, 2001.

Lawry S, McIntosh A, Rao S. *Critical Appraisal for Psychiatrists*. Edinburgh: Churchill Livingstone, 2000.

Puri B, Hall A. *Revision Notes in Psychiatry*, 2nd edn. London: Arnold/ Hodder Education, 2004.